S0-BSX-102

MANAGING TEENAGE PREGNANCY

James E. Allen

with Deborah Bender

MANAGING TEENAGE PREGNANCY

Access to Abortion, Contraception, and Sex Education

PRAEGER

PRAEGER SPECIAL STUDIES • PRAEGER SCIENTIFIC

Library of Congress Cataloging in Publication Data

Allen, James Edward.
   Managing teenage pregnancy.

   Bibliography: p.
   Includes index.
   1. Pregnancy, Adolescent--United States. 2. Sex
instruction for girls. 3. Abortion--United States.
4. Contraception. I. Bender, Deborah, joint author.
II. Title.
HQ759.4.A4   362.7   79-89009
ISBN 0-03-053991-9

Published in 1980 by Praeger Publishers
CBS Educational and Professional Publishing
A Division of CBS, Inc.
521 Fifth Avenue, New York, New York 10017 U.S.A.

© 1980 by Praeger Publishers

0123456789   038   987654321

Printed in the United States of America

Dedicated to

Moye W. Freymann and Sager C. Jain

All my friends are not the kind,
I think, to be pregnant.

A 14-year-old
Southern City eighth grader

FOREWORD by

J. Richard Udry

Adolescent pregnancy is not new under the sun. Historical and anthropological data confirm its frequency at other times in our own history, and in other societies today. But pregnancy on a large scale in the United States is a phenomenon dating from about the mid-1950s. The reason for this increase in the last half of the century is clear: more and more unmarried adolescents are involved in sexual intercourse at younger and younger ages in each subsequent birth cohort. Since 1960 the sexual involvement of adolescents at younger ages has accelerated.

Adolescent childbearing has unfortunate consequences for everyone involved. It is unfortunate for the offspring, because they suffer from higher mortality and morbidity and generally experience restricted opportunity in life. It is unfortunate for the young parents because it hobbles their futures. It is unfortunate for the whole society: the rest of us pick up much of the cost of rearing such children, and all of us suffer when children face adverse circumstances and do not reach their potential as contributors to society.

It is clear that our society is not prepared to make its peace with widespread adolescent parenthood. Nor is it able to reverse the trend toward early sexual involvement. The present volume explores the public response of two communities to a widespread problem. If you cannot prevent adolescent sexual activity, and you do not want to encourage early marriage, and you do not think adolescent childbearing is good for adolescents or the society, what do you do? This book contrasts what happens in a community that does very little with one that tries to come to grips with the problem. It shows that an organized program to prevent early pregnancies may be successful.

Community leaders concerned with the problems of young people should find in this book an optimistic message. Although it chronicles the attitudes and program experience in only two places, and therefore, does not purport to be the definitive treatise on the national problem, the book does present a concrete program that any community can manage, and that holds promise for success. As such it merits national attention.

Director, Carolina Population Center

PREFACE

In this book we report a study of two U.S. communities' efforts to manage pregnancies among their adolescents. The research was sponsored by the Ford Foundation through a population studies grant to the University of North Carolina at Chapel Hill; it began in March 1976.

The teenagers in one community are three times more successful in controlling their fertility than the teenagers in the other community. We believe our results demonstrate that it is primarily the policy makers and service providers in these two communities who through their day-to-day decisions determine whether the teenagers in their community have high or low rates of pregnancies, abortions, and births. The teenagers themselves obviously have a role, but it is the adults in their community who make the rules and succeed or fail in helping their children learn to manage their own sexuality. We believe that it is not just by chance or the result of rural and urban differences that adults in one community have taken a number of policy decisions that have enabled their teenagers to manage their fertility three times more successfully (using the criteria for success developed by the U.S. Department of Health, Education and Welfare's Center for Disease Control in Atlanta).

When we selected the two study sites, we had little idea that the communities would show two startlingly consistent and different approaches—one successful and the other unsuccessful—toward managing adolescent fertility.

During the years 1970-77 both communities had well-established, active, publicly funded family planning programs. Despite the presence of these well-established programs serving teenagers in both communities, Figure P.1 shows that over the period in question, the birthrates for both black and white teenagers trended consistently downward in the community practicing our recommended policies (Southern City). Figure P.1 also shows that during the same years birthrates remained consistently high, especially for black teenagers, in the community rejecting our recommended policies (Farmville). Documentation and discussion of why one community is failing and one community is succeeding in reducing teenage pregnancies appear throughout the book.

The undesirable consequences of early childbearing have been extensively documented in the literature, and we do not repeat them in this book. Instead, we focus on the ways the adult populations

FIGURE P.1

Percent Deviation above Desired Birthrate, Females Aged 15 to 19, Farmville and Southern City, 1970–77

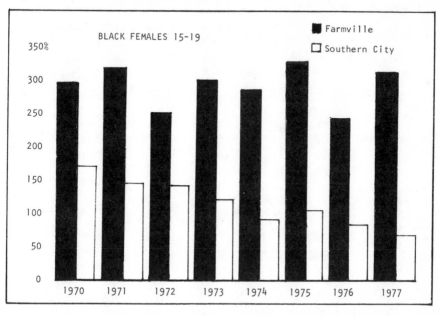

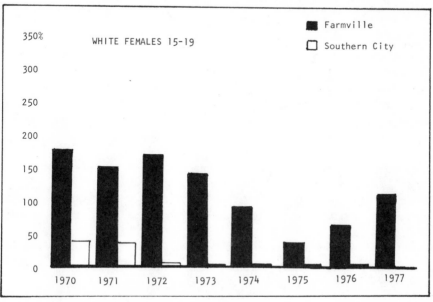

Source: Constructed by the author.

in two U.S. communities with certain characteristics are going about the task of helping their children learn to manage their fertility. We use the American Public Health Association guidelines for community management of adolescent fertility as the primary criteria with which to judge success and failure.

The data on these two communities are placed in a state and national context in order to help readers decide what relevance our findings and conclusions may have on their own beliefs about how U.S. communities can help their teenagers learn to manage their own fertility.

ACKNOWLEDGMENTS

The Carolina Population Center and the Department of Health Administration in the School of Public Health at the University of North Carolina at Chapel Hill made this research possible through awarding Ford Foundation funds and allowing a reduced work load for the principal investigators. Careful work by the eight research assistants and interviewers—Rankin Whittington, Cecil Tickamyer, Bill Brown, Sally Brown, Bill Trent, Alison Woomert, Sasha Loring, and Jane Waddell—made a project of this scope feasible and manageable. Patient and efficient typists—Patricia Mitchell, Debbie Ussery, Carolyn Strange, and Gail Thompson—endured the constant revisions with grace. Richard Udry, Carolina Population Center director, and Estelle Cardona, his assistant, marshaled the resources of the Population Center to bring many parts of the effort into focus. That the manuscript came together in an acceptable form is due to unending hours of help and encouragement from Lunn Igoe, editor for the Carolina Population Center.

Overall research design, field supervision, and the personal interviews of policy makers and service providers in Farmville were the responsibility of the senior author. The junior author, who conducted the interviews with the teenage mothers in Farmville, wrote Chapter 7 and the portions of the manuscript focusing on the teenage mothers in the two communities. Contacting and interviewing teenage mothers to ask all kinds of questions about a pregnancy most teenagers had never expected required the sensitive interviewing skills that Deborah Bender possesses. Often, when she interviewed, she received more than just the answers to her questions. Noticing the interviewer's own pregnancy, the adolescents were quick to augment the stories of their pregnancies and birth experiences with words of advice to the mother-to-be.

And to our spouses we owe a debt of thanks for their patience in the face of our frustrations, their encouragement after long days in the field, and their continued interest in our research problem and its possible solutions.

CONTENTS

LIST OF TABLES

xix

LIST OF FIGURES

MANAGING
TEENAGE
PREGNANCY

1

OVERVIEW OF THE STUDY

This study reports efforts by two U.S. communities, one urban and the other rural, to manage fertility among their adolescents. The urban community, which we will call Southern City, is a useful model for persons and communities interested in the successful management of fertility among teenage students in junior and senior high schools. The rural community, which we call Farmville, offers useful clues to understanding why so many U.S. communities are ineffective and unsuccessful in their efforts to help teenagers, especially the younger ones, manage their sexuality. Decisions in these two communities to help or not to help teenagers control their fertility are based on the values we found there.

In the following pages we measure and report positive and negative impacts on the lives of teenagers that flow out of the value orientations of the key service providers and policy makers in Farmville and Southern City. We also present state and national perspectives on the policy makers' views in these two communities.

We believe that the recent dramatic rises in the numbers of births and abortions among teenagers are largely preventable. The scientific knowledge and the types of community resources necessary to improve teenagers' ability to manage their fertility are already available. Teenage pregnancy is, in the final analysis, a problem of social values. It is the two differing value orientations in our study communities that lead to the unsuccessful Farmville and the successful Southern City efforts to help teenagers manage their sexuality.

NEED FOR A NEW CULTURAL RESPONSE

> I was kinda young when I got pregnant. I didn't think
> I would get pregnant. The doctor, he didn't know if I
> could carry it. He was really worried.
>
> > Fifteen-year-old mother
> > of a hydrocephalic child

Teenagers from upper- and middle-income families, both white and black, are becoming pregnant, obtaining abortions, and giving birth in unprecedented numbers. As knowledge of the extent of early childbearing among U.S. teenagers has grown, it has become apparent that all groups in our population are affected. The large numbers of babies being born to younger teenagers are increasingly being understood as a health problem affecting significant numbers of adolescents, their children, and their families in virtually all communities in the United States.

Early childbearing is now a problem for the entire nation. For various reasons, many of which are poorly understood, sexual mores have changed among younger people in the United States, largely through the breakdown of community mores previously believed capable of controlling adolescent fertility. Reliance on moral teachings proscribing nonmarital sex no longer controls fertility among adolescents. Clearly, for whatever reasons, recent trends in sexual behavior among U.S. teenagers have rendered traditional efforts to manage adolescent sexuality ineffective, forcing our society into a search for a new cultural response to the problem of high adolescent fertility rates. What is not clear is what the new cultural response will be. It will evolve and establish itself over a period of decades.

POLICIES FOR U.S. COMMUNITIES

In the early 1970s the American Public Health Association (APHA) recognized that no policies for care exist to guide communities interested in reducing the number of pregnancies among their junior and senior high school students.

Guides for U.S. communities had not been developed, in part, because our communities have never adequately recognized that pregnancy among adolescents is a public health problem of major proportions. Communities have not understood that pregnant teenagers, especially younger ones, usually do not know how to find help and usually are not successful in gaining access to the health care system.

Believing that the evidence indicates that communities wish to help adolescents manage their sexuality, but are uncertain about how to do so, the APHA called together a task force of representatives from numerous sections of its membership and professional groups beyond the APHA. The task force was to develop policies that concerned communities could employ to reduce the teenage pregnancy rate, especially among junior and senior high school students. The policies were to be based on accepted practice, scientific documentation, and the judgments of leading health professionals. Over a period of five years, through constant revisions and reviews by numerous national organizations, they were evolved. The resulting policies represent the best thinking of health professionals who are concerned about the high rates of pregnancies among adolescents, especially younger adolescents.

Some of the APHA policy proposals are relatively noncontroversial, unlikely to stir up opposition in communities where they are used. For example, nearly everyone can agree that "early and consistent prenatal care should be available and accessible for those young women continuing their pregnancies to term." On the other hand, a policy of making contraceptives and abortions available free and without parental consent in every community could easily arouse opposition.

The following policies are the primary focus of this research report:

1. Adolescents are individuals and should be treated with respect and a nonjudgmental attitude, in an atmosphere of privacy and confidentiality.

2. Adolescents must be provided access to sex and family life education, contraceptive advice and treatment, pregnancy testing, abortion, and prenatal/postpartun care without parental consent.

3. Adequate financial support should be available so that access to services is not restricted.

4. Provisions should be made for the early detection of pregnancy in adolescent women, and information concerning the availability of this service should be emphasized.

5. All alternatives for dealing with the pregnancy must be presented as viable solutions.

6. An interdisciplinary, comprehensive approach should be used in dealing with adolescent pregnancy.

All 15 of the policies are presented in Appendix A.

The intent is that U.S. communities use these policies to manage adolescent fertility. Four basic questions immediately arise:

1. To what extent are the needs identified in the policies already being met?

2. How would the public and community, state, and federal policy makers react to the idea of adopting these policies?

3. What are the views of the teenagers who are already using these services?

4. If these policies are adopted by communities, will they actually lead to successful community management of adolescent fertility rates?

This research project answers the four questions by intensively studying two U.S. communities. Our study includes the administrative hierarchy, members of the community, and the consumers of health services—the teenagers themselves.

It is important to find answers to these questions because the number of pregnancies occurring among younger adolescent women is reaching crisis proportions. Knowledge about how local policy makers, service providers, teenagers, and the general public would react to implementing these policies in their communities is important to any large-scale effort to implement them on the local level. These policies or very similar ones must be put into action if teenagers are to be provided with the help they need to manage their sexuality.

2

RESEARCH METHODOLOGY

SCOPE OF THE RESEARCH FOCUS

Figure 2.1 is a simplified schematic representation of an overview of attitudes and beliefs that we believe are related to the American Public Health Association (APHA) policies for managing adolescent pregnancies. At least four levels influence adolescents' decisions
leading to the occurrence or prevention of early childbearing; the individual decision maker, the local community context in which the individual makes the decision, the state and its network of policies, and
the federal context with its influences on policies.

Although the state and federal contexts are important, the primary focus of our study is the local level. In the structure of the
U.S. health care network, local communities implement whatever
policies community decision makers choose as best for the community.
State and federal influences are usually present and have an important
impact on local policies; nevertheless, it is the local community within
which individuals grow up and make daily decisions that lead to or
avert early childbearing.

Following is a summary of how our study uses the four levels
in our research methodology.

Level 1: The individual. Using three instruments, we interviewed a sample of teenagers who gave birth in 1976 in the two study
communities. We wanted to gain a detailed picture of their experience.
The interviewer asked the teenagers to recount details of their pregnancies: why they became pregnant, how they first discovered they
were pregnant, the people with whom they discussed their pregnancy,
the people they avoided telling of their pregnancy, the pattern of contraceptive use they had adopted, and their own reaction on discovering

FIGURE 2.1

Schematic Representation of Four Levels of Attitudes and Beliefs Related to the APHA Policies for Management of Adolescent Pregnancies

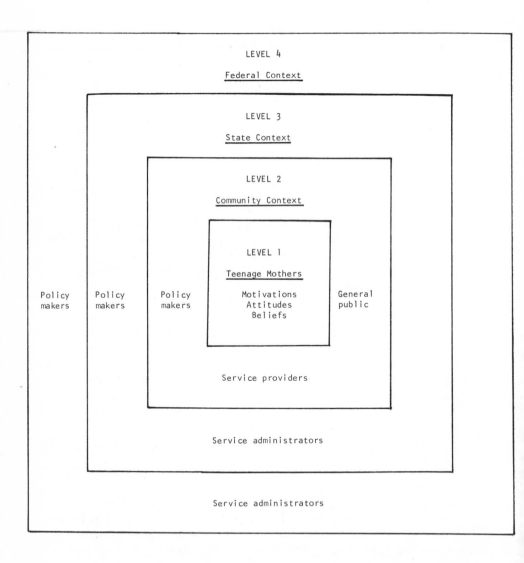

Source: Constructed by the author.

their pregnancy. We also tried to find out what health care services the girls used and when they availed themselves of these services. Finally, the teenagers interviewed were asked to make recommendations about how their care might have been improved.

Level 2: Local community context. We studied policy makers, service providers, teenagers, and a random sample of the general public to ascertain, first, their understanding of the care network for managing adolescent pregnancies currently functioning in the community and, second, to understand their beliefs and attitudes toward the APHA policies for preventing and managing pregnancies among adolescents.

Level 3: State context. Policy makers and human services administrators, who on the state level represented the same decision-making groups we studied at the local level, completed our questionnaire.

Level 4: Federal context. Policy makers and human services administrators who represented the same policy-making groups and administrators already studied at the state and local levels also completed our questionnaire.

At each level of the study, the one primary criterion was, Does the person/group influence decision making about the management of adolescent fertility in the community under study? The teenagers, who are the ultimate decision makers, are the initial focus of the study. The rationale for including policy makers and service providers in the study is discussed in greater detail below.

CRITERIA FOR SELECTING STUDY SITES

Choice of Communities

The examination and evaluation of health care services and the patterns of their use by pregnant adolescents are necessary and preliminary steps in the development of any intervention strategy. Our study focuses on two communities within one of the several hundred local health planning agencies in the nationwide system established by Public Law 93-641, the National Health Planning and Resource Development Act of 1974.

There were four criteria for choosing the two communities in the study:

1. Presence of black population,
2. Availability of one rural and one urban community,
3. Absence of special or unusual programs for managing adolescent pregnancies, and

    4. One community characterized by a relatively high rate of
adolescent childbearing, one by a relatively low rate.

    The communities having the ideal characteristics were selected
from a multicounty area served by a health systems agency in North
Carolina. This area includes three large and three small urban areas
and at least six highly rural counties, thus providing a good range of
possible study sites. The region is a mix of industrial, research,
and communications-oriented areas, with heavily agricultural areas
short distances away. The two sites chosen will be referred to as
Farmville and Southern City. Although place and personal names are
fictitious, the data in this report are accurate for each study site.
Southern City has a metropolitan area population of 270,000. The city
is a communications and industrial center for the region. Farmville
is a highly agricultural county with a total population of nearly 33,000.
It is progressive, seeking to attract outside business and industry to
supplement its agricultural economy. It has been relatively successful in this effort in recent years. Most businesses, however, are
still related to farming. Extensive additional data on these two communities will be given when describing their family planning programs,
sex education efforts, and adolescent fertility management efforts.
At this point, let us examine the two communities in terms of meeting the four criteria set up for inclusion in the study.

    Criterion 1: Representative number of black residents. Both
communities have a black population larger than the proportion of
blacks in the U.S. population. The Farmville population is 28 percent black (7,825 blacks and 25,898 whites as of July 1, 1976); the
Southern City population has 61,840 blacks and 207,744 whites (29.7
percent black).
    Criterion 2: Urban-rural representativeness. Farmville County
is highly agricultural, has no urban center, and is sufficiently far
from urban centers to have its own integrity as a farm-oriented community. It is small geographically and functions as a single community with a town of about 12,000 located in its geographical center.
Southern City has a full range of socioeconomic groups and areas, including a central city established long enough to be experiencing urban blight. Large concentrations of blacks are within the central city
area. Predominantly white suburbs surround the central city.
    Criterion 3: Normal experience in controlling adolescent fer-
tility. In the early 1970s a small, federally sponsored sex education
program was undertaken in Southern City by a concerned physician
from a nearby university. Aside from this effort, completed in the
mid-1970s, there have been no major interventions of outside funding
or leadership efforts in the two communities. That is, the sex edu-

cation efforts in both communities and the network of care set up to provide for family planning, abortion services, and other adolescent fertility-related programmatic efforts have been undertaken essentially with local funds and initiative. In Farmville there has been a federally funded family planning program for several years. The funds have come to the county through a routine flow from Washington to the regional office in Atlanta, thence to the family planning office in Raleigh, and finally to the regional Council of Governments, which has distributed the funds to counties in its area, including Farmville. Southern City has a history of somewhat less-than-normal dependency on outside funds for services related to adolescent fertility management. The Health Department has for some years sponsored an extensive family planning program relying almost exclusively on county funds. Regular bureaucratic channels have been employed in efforts to deal with preventing and managing adolescent pregnancies.

Criterion 4: High and low rates of adolescent childbearing. Table 2.1 gives the number, range, and ratios of births to women 17 and younger in Farmville, Southern City, and the multicounty health systems agency area in 1975. Farmville had a higher-than-average percentage of total births to women 17 or younger, according to calculations based on the number of births and total number of females aged 10 to 17. In the multicounty area Farmville had the fourth highest percentage of births to women 17 or younger (13.1 percent). The percentage of total births to black women 17 or younger (25.9 percent) was the highest in the multicounty area. The ratio of white to black births among women 17 and younger was one to six—one white birth for every six black births—the second highest in the health systems agency area.

Conversely, Southern City had the second-from-lowest percentage of births to women 17 and younger (6.8 percent) in the health systems agency area. The Southern City pregnancy rate for whites aged 17 and younger (3.5 percent) was third lowest in the health systems agency area. The rate for blacks aged 17 and younger was the fourth from lowest.

In 1975, Farmville registered 20 legitimate and 45 out-of-wedlock births (65); Southern City showed 87 legal and 158 out-of-wedlock births (245) to women 17 and under. In Farmville the mothers' ages ranged from 14 to 17; in Southern City, from 13 to 17.

For a study community with a relatively high rate of early childbearing, Farmville County is a good choice. The percentage of births to whites was twice that in Southern City and moderately above the average for the multicounty area. The percentage of births to blacks was quite high, the highest in the multicounty area (25.9 percent). Southern City was also a good choice because the percentage of births to white women 17 and younger was half that of Farmville and lower than the average for the multicounty area.

TABLE 2.1

Statistics on Births to Women Aged 17 and Younger, Farmville,
Southern City, and Multicounty Health Systems Agency Area, 1975

	Farmville	Southern City	Multi-county Area	Range (percent)
Total				
Total births	498	3,578	9,933	5.4
17 and younger births	65	345	877	to
Percent	13.1	6.8	8.8	14.5
White				
Total births	322	2,463	6,134	2.2
17 and younger births	22	87	288	to
Percent	6.6	3.5	4.7	9.0
Nonwhite				
Total births	166	1,115	3,799	12.5
17 and younger births	43	158	589	to
Percent	25.9	14.2	15.5	25.9

Ratio of White to Nonwhite Births	
Farmville	1:6.2
Southern City	1:5.0
Multicounty area	1:3.9

Source: North Carolina Department of Human Resources, Public Health Statistics Branch, 1975 Babybook, N.C. Resident Births
(Raleigh: Department of Human Resources, 1975).

State Characteristics

Because the North Carolina experience seems reasonably typical
of other states, we felt no need to seek a study site outside the state
in which we were already located. Several comparisons between North
Carolina and other states are given below.

North Carolina has made a consistent effort to provide human
services to its citizens. The history of family planning in the state
dates back to 1937, when the first family planning clinic was opened.
Nearly all of the state's 100 counties had family planning clinics
shortly after the end of World War II. In terms of progress in social
services and family planning, the subsequent years have been typical
for a mid-Atlantic state.

Share of Early Childbearing

North Carolina has a comparatively high share of early childbearing. In terms of percentage of births to females 19 and younger

TABLE 2.2

Percentage of Total Births to Females Aged 19 and Younger for
Each State and HEW Region, United States, 1974

State and Region	Percent	State and Region	Percent
Region I		Region VI	
Connecticut	13	Arkansas	26
Maine	18	Louisiana	24
Massachusetts	13	New Mexico	21
New Hampshire	14	Oklahoma	24
Rhode Island	15	Texas	22
Vermont	16	Region VII	
Region II		Iowa	16
New Jersey	14	Kansas	19
New York	13	Missouri	21
Region III		Nebraska	15
Delaware	21	Region VIII	
District of Columbia	28	Colorado	18
Maryland	18	Montana	18
Pennsylvania	17	North Dakota	15
Virginia	20	South Dakota	18
West Virginia	23	Utah	12
Region IV		Wyoming	19
Alabama	26	Region IX	
Florida	24	Arizona	20
Georgia	25	California	17
Kentucky	25	Hawaii	15
Mississippi	29	Nevada	20
North Carolina	25	Region X	
South Carolina	25	Alaska	16
Tennessee	25	Idaho	16
Region V		Oregon	17
Illinois	19	Washington	16
Indiana	22		
Michigan	19		
Minnesota	13		
Ohio	20		
Wisconsin	15		

Note: HEW = Department of Health, Education and Welfare.

Source: National Center for Health Statistics, Division of Analysis, "Natality Statistics," mimeographed (Washington, D.C.: Office of the Assistant Secretary for Health, 1976).

TABLE 2.3

Number of Births by Mother's Age and Race, North Carolina, 1974

Mother's Age	Total	White	Black
Under 15	511	161	348
15 to 19	20,765	11,592	8,729
20 to 24	29,819	20,596	3,585
25 to 29	21,733	17,198	4,014
30 to 34	8,241	6,343	1,682
35 to 39	2,562	1,735	753
40 to 44	587	348	211
45 to 49	26	16	10
Total	84,244	57,803	24,332

Note: "Total" column excludes 2.5 percent classified as "other."

Source: Prepared by Maternal and Child Health Studies Project of Information Sciences Research Institute, Washington, D.C., 1976.

in 1974, it was well above the U.S. average of 19 percent. As Table 2.2 shows, 3 states had a higher percentage, 4 had the same percentage, and 42 had lower percentages of births to females aged 19 and younger.

In North Carolina in 1974, there were 511 births to females younger than 15 and 20,756 births to females aged 15 to 19. With total births of 84,244, births to females under 20 accounted for 25 percent of all births. Numerically fewer births occurred to blacks. However, when the ratio of whites and blacks in the total population was taken into account, the fertility rate for 1974 in North Carolina (see Table 2.3) was 59 per 1,000 for blacks aged 13 to 17, in contrast with 28,9 for whites.

Comparisons of Abortions Obtained

To allow the reader to draw further conclusions as to the suitability of North Carolina as a state for study and its position relative to other states, Table 2.4 gives 1968-72 birth and fertility data for selected states, and Table 2.5 gives 1974 abortion data in selected

TABLE 2.4

Fertility Rates for Total, White, and Other Teenagers, Selected States and District of Columbia, 1968–72

State	Births			Fertility Rate		
	Total	White	Other	Total	White	Other
California	98,395	75,005	23,390	21.3	18.4	42.5
District of Columbia	8,918	388	8,530	57.9	21.7	62.6
Florida	50,443	25,719	24,724	33.4	21.6	76.5
Georgia	45,017	20,668	24,349	39.6	26.7	67.0
Iowa	10,564	9,804	760	15.2	14.3	70.1
Kentucky	25,045	20,563	4,482	31.8	28.5	69.3
Massachusetts	14,162	11,592	2,570	11.0	9.4	51.2
New York	63,665	36,073	27,592	15.8	10.5	47.2
North Carolina	42,658	20,320	22,338	33.8	28.9	59.1
South Carolina	24,077	10,161	13,916	34.9	24.3	51.3

Note: The fertility rate is the rate per 1,000 females, aged 13 to 17, based on 1968–73 birth data and the population of females aged 13 to 17 in 1970.

Source: National Center for Health Statistics, Division of Analysis, "Natality Statistics," mimeographed (Washington, D.C.: Office of the Assistant Secretary for Health, October 1976), table 6.

TABLE 2.5

Percentage of Reported Legal Abortions Obtained by Teenagers,
Selected States, 1974

	Age 15		Ages 15 to 19	
State	Number	Percent	Number	Percent
California	1,973	1.5	45,409	33.4
District of Columbia	369	1.6	5,999	26.4
Georgia	435	2.0	7,053	32.0
Kentucky	199	4.0	1,898	37.7
New York	1,715	1.1	41,202	25.5
City	1,219	1.0	28,439	23.5
Upstate	496	1.2	12,763	31.4
North Carolina	388	2.4	5,791	35.2
South Carolina	76	2.0	1,186	31.5
South Dakota	13	0.8	588	36.7
Tennessee	150	2.0	2,653	35.8
Virginia	328	2.3	5,205	36.2

Source: U.S., Department of Health, Education and Welfare,
Public Health Service, Abortion Surveillance 1974 (Atlanta: Center
for Disease Control, 1976), table 6, p. 20.

TABLE 2.6

Number and Percent of Reported Legal Abortions, by Age, United
States, 1974

Age	Number	Percent
15	8,630	1.5
15 to 19	177,196	30.0
20 to 24	180,735	31.4
25 to 29	102,917	17.9
30 to 34	57,046	9.9
35 to 39	30,689	5.3
40	11,873	2.1
Unknown	5,073	0.9
Total	574,159	100.0

Source: U.S., Department of Health, Education and Welfare,
Public Health Service, Abortion Surveillance 1974 (Atlanta: Center
for Disease Control, 1976), table 6, p. 20.

states. The reported rate of legal abortions to teenagers under 15 in North Carolina was 2.4 percent, (Table 2.5), compared with a national average of 1.5 percent (Table 2.6). The percentage of North Carolina abortions performed on teenagers 15 to 19 was 35.2 percent, also above the national average of 30 percent. Thus, while North Carolina was 6 percent above the national average in births to females aged 19 and younger—a worse-than-average record by 6 percent—37.6 percent of its teenagers were able to obtain wanted abortions (see Table 2.5) compared with the national average of 31.6 percent (see Table 2.6).

Federal-Level Characteristics

We have discussed the criteria on which we chose the two local communities and the characteristics of the state in the study. The rationale for including the federal level in this study parallels that of including state-level decision makers: the context of community decision making extends to Washington in a more nearly one-to-one relationship than might at first seem likely. It is true that decisions by Congress and the president are four or more administrative layers away from everyday decision making in Farmville and Southern City. The time lag is sometimes lengthy, but the laws, executive decisions, and regulations at the levels of Washington and the federal region (Atlanta) do get passed through the state capital in Raleigh, and influence the options available to local communities in their decision making about the management of adolescent fertility.

In the end, it really makes little difference that the decision-making time lag exists. The effect on decision making in local communities is no less direct. Also, there are times when decisions by the president and Congress do have a one-to-one, direct, and immediate impact on local community decision making. For example, a 1977 decision by Congress to ban the use of Medicaid funds for abortions had direct and immediate effects on local communities. The county commissioners and city councilmen in both Farmville and Southern City were faced the day after the funding cutoff with a decision on whether to use county or city tax dollars to fill the gap left by the federal decision. The state later decided to continue to fund Medicaid abortions with state tax money. The necessity for decision and the impact of the Washington decision in this case were simultaneously transmitted to the federal regional offices, the states, and the counties and cities. In sum, the administrative distance between Washington and the local community may seem to be great at times, but the omnipresence and continuing impact of federal decisions,

whatever the time lag, keep the links between Washington and communities like Farmville and Southern City strong.

We have described the criteria by which we chose Farmville,
Southern City, and the state of North Carolina for our study. We turn
now to a description of the people and groups we included in this study
at each level.

RESULTS OBTAINED

The four levels of attitudes and beliefs related to the APHA
policies for managing adolescent pregnancy appeared in Figure 2.1.
Each of these four levels is discussed here in terms of how it contrib-
utes to an understanding of the overall problem of managing teenage
pregnancies. (Our test instruments appear in Appendix B.) A detailed description of results obtained in each category, methodology
used, and information on our pretests and follow-up procedures appear in Appendix C.

Level 1: The Teenage Mother

The adolescents we interviewed are selected from among the
cohort of teenagers who gave birth in 1976 in Southern City and Farmville. In Farmville an attempt was made to contact each of the 76
girls aged 17 and under who delivered in 1976. A representative
sample of 40 teenagers in Southern City was selected from more than
230 who gave birth. This sample was balanced for age and race
against the Farmville sample—35 teenage mothers were successfully
interviewed in Farmville; 36 interviews were completed in Southern
City.

We are very conscious that an important segment of teenagers
served has been left out of our study: those who received abortions
during 1976. In order to minimize the gap left by not being able to
identify and interview those persons because of confidentiality laws,
we thoroughly researched the abortion data for both communities during that calendar year. Thus, while we are unable to present interviews with the individuals who obtained abortions in 1976, we have
thorough data on the number and geographical locations of teenage
abortions in the two communities by race and age. The data enable
us to have reasonable estimates of the frequency of abortions during
1976, as well as information on the women who gave birth.

Another group important to the service system is those teenagers who sought and received contraceptive assistance during 1976
at either a private physician's office or the public health clinic. Data
by age and race on these persons were obtained through interviews

with the service providers and from information at the family planning clinic.

Level 2: The Community Context

We interviewed representatives of every group of persons who were thought to have some influence on the management of adolescent fertility in the two communities. To accomplish this we divided the community into four groups: the general public, policy makers, service providers, and educators. A random sample of the entire general public of the two communities was obtained through a mailed questionnaire. We sought a completed sample of at least 200 persons from the general public in each community. Of those who were mailed questionnaires, 40 percent responded in each community, yielding 234 usable questionnaires in Farmville and 215 in Southern City. The race, sex, income, education, religion, and age distributions of the respondents and the general population are reasonably similar. (The mostly small differences, such as an underrepresentation of persons in their twenties, are discussed in detail in Appendix C.) In Farmville we personally interviewed major proportions of the policy makers, service providers, and educators. In Southern City, where sheer numbers posed a problem, we used a combination of interviews and questionnaires mailed to them.

We defined the policy group as including all members of boards that had any relationship to decision making in the area of teenage pregnancy, including all city councilmen and county commissioners, the health board, the social services board, the mental health board, the school board, and school administrators. Ministerial Association members and other ministers were interviewed as members of the policy-making group. Ministers also have counseling roles that we studied.

In Farmville we sought to interview all these policy-making persons. We interviewed 72 Farmville policy makers, representing all but six members of the above-mentioned governmental bodies and boards. Those six either were away on vacation or could not be reached after five attempts. In Southern City, from each board or governmental body we identified the three members judged by their peers as knowledgeable about adolescent pregnancies and interviewed a total of 42 policy makers. All persons interviewed were asked to name other persons in the community whom they thought had influence on community decisions about the prevention and management of adolescent pregnancies. We interviewed a group of these named influentials in each community.

Service providers were defined as persons providing any kind of service directly related to the prevention or treatment of pregnancies among adolescents in the community. In this category we interviewed medical doctors; other medical professionals; staffs of the health, social services, and mental health departments; pharmacists; and school counselors. We interviewed 36 service providers in Farmville and 33 in Southern City.

Level 3: The State Context

At the state and federal levels we replicated to the degree feasible a study of the persons and groups equivalent to those studied at the community level. Under policy makers we included the executive branch, all state senators, and all state representatives. In addition to the legislators and the executive branch, we surveyed all judges in the state down through the district court judges, which included those for Farmville and Southern City—54 percent of the North Carolina state senators and 62 percent of the state representatives participated in our study; 63 percent of all judges down through the district courts participated, including six of the seven North Carolina Supreme Court judges.

In North Carolina the state-level equivalents of the local service providers (with the exception of the pharmacists) are the human services administrators of each of the state-level departments that are the counterparts of the community departments—for example, the Health Department, the Youth Services Department, and the regional offices of the Department of Human Resources (which includes all the above-mentioned departments). All of the 58 top state human services administrators asked to participate in the study did so.

Level 4: The Federal Context

The federal equivalents of community and state policy makers, human services administrators, and educators were included in the study universe. All U.S. senators and representatives were sent the questionnaire.

Most congressmen responded that by policy they do not participate in any mail surveys. A total of 11 members of the U.S. Senate and 72 members of the U.S. House of Representatives participated. Human services administrators included were in the Public Health Service and its Mental Health Administration, the Social Security Administration, the National Institutes of Health, the Office of Education, and the Department of Health, Education and Welfare regional offices.

Often there were no exact equivalents at the state and federal levels for the local agencies included in the study, but to the degree possible we included the actual direct equivalents. Forty-one (76 percent) of our sample of top U.S. Department of Health, Education and Welfare administrators participated, including eight of the ten regional directors.

DEVELOPMENT OF INSTRUMENTS AND PRETESTS

The development of instruments for this study was less complicated than normal for a study of such magnitude, since the policies that are the heart of the research focus were painstakingly developed by the APHA over a five-year period. Each policy was reviewed, edited, rewritten, and modified dozens of times by persons and groups within and outside the APHA. Our job was to put these policies into a format that would allow us to test them among the various persons and groups within the study population.

We rephrased each into a simple, neutrally stated policy. The original policy ideas were cast in a hortatory style that was unacceptable for our purposes. In order to allow the full range of attitudes to be included, we added the following items to the original policies:

1. Allowing information about sex only to persons over 18,
2. Refusing abortions to anyone under 18,
3. Requesting pregnant girls to leave school before the fifth month of pregnancy,
4. Encouraging unmarried teenagers to accept responsibility for pregnancy by having the child,
5. Emphasizing the teaching that sexual union outside of marriage is a sin,
6. Keeping sex education out of the schools, and
7. Restricting contraceptives to persons over 18.

There were several purposes to be accomplished by adding these items. First, it was essential to develop a questionnaire that allowed all respondents, no matter where their opinion fell along a continuum, to find items with which they could agree and that expressed their opinion. For example, if individuals were strongly in favor of not providing any information or help for teenagers under the age of 18, without these seven additions there would be few if any items to which they could respond favorably. An additional reason for including the seven items was to allow the researchers to check for consistency of responses, which would provide a measure of the reliability of the study instrument by measuring respondents' beliefs and attitudes on both the positive and the negative dimensions of the same issue.

TABLE 2.7

Instruments Developed for the Study: Title, Subject, Content, Method of Administration, and Category of Respondents

Form	Title	Subject and Content	Administration	Respondents
A	Study of Adolescent Pregnancies (short form)	20 questions covering attitudes and beliefs about the 15 APHA standards	Mail, interview	All respondents at all levels
B	Study of Adolescent Pregnancies (long form)	20 questions on the 15 APHA standards plus 13 questions on what teenage girls do when they suspect pregnancy	Mail, interview	All community-level respondents
C	Medical Service Providers	14 questions probing medical services to teenagers seeking fertility control help	Interview	Medical providers in two communities
D	Ministers	11 questions probing ministers' counseling practices	Interview	Ministers in two communities
E	Counselors	13 questions probing counseling techniques used in the community	Interview	Counselors in two communities
F	Pharmacists	6 questions probing pharmacists' practices	Interview	Pharmacists in two communities
G	School Study	8 questions probing school practices	Mail	Educators throughout state
H	Personal Response Question Set	24 questions probing teenage mothers' beliefs and experiences	Interview	Teenage women who gave birth in 1976 in two communities
I	Heuristic Elicitation Question Frame	16 questions probing teenage mothers' use of the care network	Interview	Teenage women who gave birth in 1976 in two communities

Note: See Appendix B for forms.

Source: Compiled by the author.

To trace the network of care available to teenagers as they saw it, a series of questions was developed to allow us to gauge what teenagers do when they suspect pregnancy. These questions were designed to let the respondent answer in her own words. This methodology allowed us to become familiar with the cultural categories defined by the adolescent. In an attempt to understand the values and motivations of pregnant teenagers, an instrument was developed to query them on their attitudes toward pregnancy and contraceptives.

In all, nine instruments were developed and used to measure beliefs and attitudes among the groups of respondents. (See Appendix B.) The title, contents, and uses for each of the nine forms appear in Table 2.7. Every person who participated in the study in any way was asked to respond to Form A, which contains the policies recommended by the APHA. Respondents at the state and national levels were asked to complete only Form A, which measures beliefs and attitudes toward the APHA policies. Educators were also asked to complete Form G. All the other forms were used for respondents in the two communities.

All study participants in the two communities except teenage mothers, for whom we used special forms, completed Form B, which contains 13 questions about what teenage girls do when they suspect pregnancy. Participants who fell into one of the specialized categories of medical service provider, minister, counselor, or pharmacist were asked to respond also to an additional specialized form. For example, a medical doctor would respond to Form B and to the specialized form for medical service providers (C). A city manager would respond to Form B only. Teenagers who gave birth in 1976 were asked in an interview situation to complete three forms: Form A; Form H, the Personal Response Question Set (a set of forced-choice questions focusing on attitudes toward contraceptive use and pregnancy); and Form I, the Heuristic Elicitation Question Frame (a set of open-ended questions that probed the teenagers' experience with the community network of care for preventing and responding to teenage pregnancies).

SUMMARY OF METHODOLOGY

A highly complex study population has been described. Its heart is the two communities. In both communities we theoretically specified the persons and groups to be surveyed. We included every person and every group that respondents mentioned during the study as having important inputs to community decision making about the prevention and treatment of pregnancies among adolescents. Many of the important nuances that will be reported in the following chapters are based on insights we gained in the interviews, as well as the aggregated and computer-processed data available in the tables and figures. Recognizing that this would be a crucial aspect of the study, the senior investigator conducted virtually all of the interviews in Farmville himself. The junior investigator conducted interviews with the Farmville teenagers who gave birth in 1976. Interviews in Southern City were conducted by staff members trained by the senior and junior investigators.

The APHA's recommended policies form the conceptual core of this research. They represent the considered judgments of health professionals on the prevention and management of pregnancies among adolescents in U.S. communities. As such they allow an interesting study in comparative values among health professionals, policy makers, and service providers at the community, state, and national levels. The rationale for choosing the two specific communities has been given, together with the basis for choosing North Carolina as a study site. Each reader must evaluate the usefulness of the criteria on which we based this study. Other criteria could have been used with equal rationality.

One follow-up letter was sent to initial nonrespondents. We did not interview nonrespondents. It was not our purpose to be able to guarantee within a narrow margin of accuracy that the respondents in our study exactly match the opinions and beliefs in the two communities. The additional time and expense involved in further pursuit of the sample universe did not seem to us to be justified.

Thus, we cannot characterize nonrespondents. We cannot, for example, say in what ways the 333 Farmville nonrespondents or the 299 Southern City nonrespondents differ from the 234 and 215 individuals who did respond. Obviously there are unknown biases introduced into our results by our being unable to characterize nonrespondents. Our decision was to guarantee that every resident of the two local communities had an equal chance of being selected for the study sample. The degrees of congruence between the profiles of the respondents and the profile of the actual community lead us to believe that we have a reasonably accurate and representative demographic profile of the general public in the two communities (see Appendix C). We feel that we have reliably measured the general trends of attitudes and beliefs among the general public in these two North Carolina communities.

What we believe we have achieved is a reasonable profile of beliefs, attitudes, and practices related to the management of adolescent pregnancies in two U.S. communities with the stated characteristics. We also believe we have useful measurements of attitudes and beliefs of a significant group of policy makers and administrators at the state and national levels on the same study dimensions. In our opinion, the participation levels of the population groups specified for study allow meaningful interpretations to be made in the following chapters. We urge the reader interested in the details of our methodology and results obtained to read Appendix C. Given the prevalence of concern about early childbearing in the United States, we believe the data produced through this research in the communities meeting our stated criteria will be relevant and useful information for future U.S. policy making in this area.

The results of our research are presented in Chapters 3 through 8, followed by conclusions and recommendations in Chapter 9. The six central chapters focus sequentially on teen access to counseling, abortion, contraceptives, prenatal care, and sex education. A wide range of information and misinformation is found to exist among the groups of study participants. In each chapter we compare what the respondents reported happening with what we believe is actually happening in Farmville and Southern City. We also report how respondents feel about adoption of the APHA policies by their own community. Finally, using several available criteria for evaluation, we present our estimates of the extent of unmet need. We identify unmet need as consisting of service gaps and value gaps, believing that new values are as crucial as better services if adolescent fertility is to be managed successfully in communities similar to Farmville and Southern City. The many recommendations for change made by respondents and our own conclusions are presented in Chapter 9.

3

TEEN "COUNSELING": TALKS WITH THEIR FRIENDS

Teen access to pregnancy tests and to counseling help in making the decision to abort or have a child are crucial matters for both young women and communities. A decision for abortion must be made within the first three months of pregnancy if an early abortion is to be obtained. Entry into prenatal care is not as time bound, but it is equally important for teenagers who choose to give birth, especially younger teenagers for whom the risks to both the mother and the infant are high. The pregnancy experiences of teenagers are an important input into a community's decisions about what needs exist for contraceptive services and sex education; so we will move from an analysis of early pregnancy services, such as access to counseling and pregnancy tests, to abortion, then to antecedent needs for contraceptive services, prenatal care, and finally to sex education. In this chapter and in Chapter 4 we report on the community impressions in the following research areas: to whom teenagers first talk and where they go for help when they first suspect pregnancy, where they can be tested for pregnancy, and what sources of counseling help they have.

TYPICAL CASES

Patti Davis (all names are fictitious), age 16, stood in a Farm-ville phone booth, crying. She dialed number after number, but hung up before anyone had a chance to answer. She was upset, confused, and at times angry. The reason? She was pregnant, and had no idea where to turn for help. Her boyfriend had left her, her parents had been separated for years and had their own problems, and friends had told her that the Public Health Department would not give contraceptives to anyone under 18. "If they wouldn't help then," Patti reasoned

24

to herself, "I could never expect them to help me now." And without any money, going to a private doctor, the only other option Patti could think of, was clearly out of the question. So she stood in the phone booth for a very long time.

Patti's situation is not that uncommon, agrees Martha Maxwell, a self-styled Farmville "health facilitator." Martha now spends many hours talking with young girls who are pregnant and do not know what to do. She has a great deal of empathy for the girls who come to talk, for she was once in the same position. She too was 16 when her first child was born. Only through trial and error and persistent questioning at each place she visited was Martha able to find prenatal health care that satisfied her needs. She realizes that most girls who become pregnant did not plan to get pregnant, and therefore do not know what is important to them in health care. What Martha is certain of, however, is that the girls she talks with are very quick to decide what they do not like about the care they receive. "They don't know how important good care is for both mother and baby. When they are dissatisfied, they don't search for an alternative. They just don't go back," she commented.

Martha's point of view is supported by birth records kept by the state. In too many instances prenatal care is started late and too few appointments are kept for anyone's peace of mind. Poor prenatal care, coupled with statistically higher rates of prematurity, low birth weight, and birth defects, makes the outcomes of adolescent pregnancy quite bleak.

Through her constant contact with pregnant teens, Martha has gathered a number of insights into the processes by which they seek care. First, she made it clear to us that very, very few of the girls who become pregnant do so intentionally. As a matter of fact, most are quite upset and confused when they realize they are pregnant. Given these circumstances, it is quite logical to assume that young teenagers who find themselves pregnant are uncertain what to do or where to go for help or advice.

One frequently used alternative is to turn first to the father of the baby, usually someone the girl calls a boyfriend. Several girls Martha knows had done that. A typical response of a boyfriend was, "Don't you go and have an abortion" or "Go ahead and have the baby." In almost all instances in both Farmville and Southern City, the male involved was in favor of maintaining the pregnancy and having the child. When it came to seeking care and making sure that care was received continuously, boyfriends were less positive in their behavior. One girl Martha had talked to said that her boyfriend was very enthusiastic about her being pregnant. He was going to provide the doctor. In the end, the girl told Martha, "He didn't do nothing about it or do nothing for it." According to the girl, it was not so much that he did not want to help, but that he did not know where to go for help. Furthermore, he did not know how to ask someone else to make suggestions about health care.

Girl friends apparently are another source of support and encouragement. Unless they are several years older than the pregnant girl, or have had an earlier pregnancy themselves, they, too, are of little help in referring a pregnant adolescent to appropriate health services.

Most often the girl's mother is the person who ultimately gets her daughter in contact with the medical care system. Girls are somewhat reluctant to talk to their mothers, though they do so more often in Farmville than in Southern City. Martha indicated that the mother often simply takes or sends her daughter to her own doctor. In instances where a private doctor is not the option, mothers send their daughters to the Health Department clinic.

Much of what Martha had to report were her impressions. She had talked to numerous girls who had lived in Farmville most of their lives and to some girls who lived in Southern City, and had heard many more of their stories through friends. Her impressions are not far from the facts as we uncovered them in this study.

This chapter and the following three chapters follow a sequence: (1) what people think is happening in their communities, which we compare with what we found is happening; (2) our estimate of the extent of unmet need (service and value gaps); and (3) how people feel about meeting the needs identified in their communities. Differences between services the people have or wish to have in their community and services called for in the American Public Health Association (APHA) policies we call value gaps.

The data gathered in this study have been organized, analyzed, and presented in tables and figures that show discrete categories and percentages to illustrate patterns of behavior in the two communities. The essence of our research, however, is in reporting the interviews with community members. The responses help the reader to realize that the people in Farmville and Southern City are real, not simply abstractions presented in a written report. From the interview responses we developed the data groupings that appear in the tables and figures—an approach that minimized introducing our own biases into the research process. Persons interviewed responded in their own words, with a minimum amount of structure imposed on them. The result, we believe, more accurately reflects the respondents' feelings and perceptions, and is especially important in our research project because there are no necessarily right or wrong answers in most of the areas we investigate. Rather, each respondent holds opinions, feelings, and biases based on an individual value system. These opinions, feelings, and biases affect the services available and their use by sexually active school-age girls.

WHAT PEOPLE REPORT IS HAPPENING
IN THEIR COMMUNITIES

> They talk to no one and hope that it hasn't happened.
> A physician member of the
> health board in Southern City

Summaries of the views of policy makers, service providers, and the general public in Farmville and Southern City on to whom a school-age girl in their community first goes to discuss a suspected pregnancy are given in Table 3.1 (see also Figure 3.1). All groups in both communities agreed consistently that about a third of the time a peer is the first person in whom the pregnant teen confides. Beyond agreeing on this one aspect, there was progressively less consistency in respondents' impressions. What is most striking is that no other category of persons was viewed as being consistently consulted, a theme that is developed throughout this chapter. Parents were mentioned about 20 percent of the time by policy makers and the general public in Farmville (16 percent and 20 percent, respectively), and significantly less frequently in Southern City (8 percent and 17 percent, respectively). The 23 teenagers in the general public samples in both communities believed that parents are never the first people the girls talk to when they suspect pregnancy. This situation would not in itself be of serious concern if teenagers had one or more sources of help available in whom their parents might have confidence.

The physician in private practice might be a reliable source of help for pregnant teens, although there was little feeling among the various respondents that the physician is a consistent source to whom teenagers first turn for help. Rural service providers felt—three times more frequently than did urban service providers (22 percent and 7 percent, respectively)—that teenagers might first talk to a private physician.

There were strong differences in perceptions between adult and teenage respondents in the two communities concerning the relative importance of the boyfriend as the person to whom girls first talk. Policy makers, service providers, and the general public were nearly unanimous in agreeing that the boyfriend is not the first person in whom the girls confide. Only 3 percent of the policy makers and 4 percent of the service providers in both communities saw the boyfriend in such a light. In actual practice the teenagers who became mothers in 1976 talked first to their boyfriends 40 percent of the time.

Service providers in both communities saw the Health Department as twice or more likely to be the first choice of teenage girls than did the policy makers and the general public. In fact, however, not one of the teenage mothers in Southern City first talked to the Health Department staff.

TABLE 3.1

Person or Other Source to Whom Young Women First Talk When
They Suspect Pregnancy: Views of Policy Makers, Service
Providers, and General Public, Farmville and Southern City, 1977
(percent)

Person or Other Source	Policy Makers		Service Providers		General Public	
	F	SC	F	SC	F	SC
Peer	35	33	30	38	31	38
Parent	16	8	6	7	20	17
Other adult	8	6	7	2	5	7
Private physician	10	10	22	7	14	7
Boyfriend	3	3	4	4	9	8
Public Health Department	3	8	13	16	6	9
Church	3	3	2	0	4	2
School	10	26	6	20	4	9
Other	12[a]	0	11[b]	4[c]	7[d]	3[e]

[a]Hospital (1), calls outside county (1), "many possibilities" (3), and "not the parents" (2).

[b]Anonymous telephone calls (1), the "hotline" telephone at the Mental Health Department (1), calls outside the county (1), Department of Social Services (1), gas station attendants (1), and "not the parents" (6).

[c]Department of Social Services (1) and "not the parents" (1).

[d]Calls outside county (6), Department of Social Services (4), Mental Health Department (1), hospitals (1), and "not the parents" (6).

[e]"Hotline" (2), call outside the area (1), Department of Social Services (2), hospital (1), and other agencies (3).

Note: F = Farmville; SC = Southern City.

Source: Compiled by the author.

FIGURE 3.1

Views of General Public on to Whom Teenagers First Talk, Compared with Reports of Teenage Mothers on What Actually Happens, Southern City, 1977

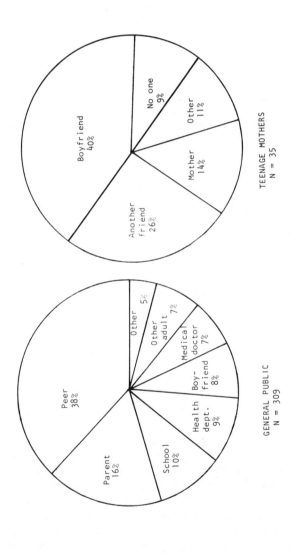

Source: Constructed by the author.

TABLE 3.2

Community Sources to Which Young Women Turn When They Suspect
Pregnancy: Views of Policy Makers, Service Providers, and
General Public, Farmville and Southern City, 1977
(percent)

Source	Policy Makers		Service Providers		General Public	
	F	SC	F	SC	F	SC
Public Health Department	19	17	26	30	23	24
Church	11	6	6	1	14	10
School	15	35	8	18	6	10
Doctor	28	7	32	2	22	10
Clinic	0	0	0	16	3	16
Department of Social Services	1	6	0	7	11	5
Hospital	1	4	0	10	0	5
Hotline	0	1	1	0	0	2
Other	25	24	27	16	21	18
Total	100	100	100	100	100	100
Number	75	62	65	55	248	309

Note: F = Farmville; SC = Southern City.

Source: Compiled by the author.

No more than 3 percent of the adult respondents in either community saw the church as a source of help for pregnant teens, and
none of the 23 teenage respondents in the general public in either
community mentioned the church.

If parents, physicians, the Public Health Department, and the
church are viewed as somewhat infrequent sources of immediate consultation, the schools might be thought of as a possible source to fill
the gaps. Farmville schools were mentioned by 10 percent of the
policy makers, 5 percent of the school providers, and 4 percent of
the general public. Teenagers in the Farmville general public sample never mentioned school personnel. Southern City respondents

mentioned schools as a source more frequently: 26 percent of the policy makers, 20 percent of the service providers, and 9 percent of the general public.

Another group of persons to whom school-age girls suspecting pregnancy might turn is other adults. But respondents felt that other adults are very seldom a teenager's first confidant: No adult group of respondents mentioned other adults more than 8 percent of the time, and the 23 teenage respondents in the general public never mentioned them at all. For example, the Department of Social Services was mentioned by only one service provider in each location, four members of the rural general public, and one member of the urban general public.

Table 3.2 reports the places and/or persons to whom respondents feel teenage girls actually turn for services. Farmville respondents mentioned the Public Health Department, churches, schools, and doctors. In contrast, the main sources of services mentioned in Southern City were the Public Health Department, schools, doctors, hospitals, abortion clinics, and the Department of Social Services, indicating a broader service pattern in Southern City.

WHAT THE RESEARCHERS FOUND

> The first thing most girls do when they find themselves pregnant is talk to their best friend, and next they seek advice from the male as to what they should do.
>
> A black school board member
> in her fifties

It is not possible to say precisely to whom teenagers suspecting pregnancy first talk and the exact places and persons to whom they turn for help. Through our research we have obtained the impressions of a large number of persons in two communities concerning what teenagers do and where they get help when they suspect pregnancy. These impressions, whether correct or incorrect, accurate or inaccurate, have an impact on the decisions about offering services and the conditions that must be met to receive them. For instance, we know the views of the county commissioners and city councilmen who make budget appropriations, the members of the various boards that establish and maintain service levels, the service providers in the various agencies and professions—such as the pharmacists and the private medical doctors—and members of the community whose feelings are perceived to influence the policy makers and the service providers. A composite picture yielding what we believe may be a reasonably useful picture of what is occurring in the two communities can be drawn from the impressions and views of these several groups.

VIEWS OF TEENAGE MOTHERS

> My boyfriend told me to go ahead and have it.
> An unmarried Southern City
> teenage mother

Thus far we have spoken of the views of policy makers, service providers, and the general public, none of whom receive any of the services we have been investigating. We were interested in being able to compare the views of those who actually received or were eligible to receive these services with the views of the policy makers and service providers. To have obtained interviews or received completed questionnaires from a random sample of schoolgirls who were sexually active or who had suspected and/or confirmed a pregnancy would have been ideal. However, we had no way of identifying those girls. We knew that an unknown number of school-age young women in the two communities do suspect a pregnancy or become pregnant each year, and we have compiled as many statistics about these events as we could find. It was not possible to obtain data from teenagers who obtained an abortion. To whom they first talk and where they go for assistance are unknown; we know only that they manage their pregnancy through obtaining an abortion.

A number of teenage schoolgirls in the two communities delivered a child during 1976. We chose to study this group because they were the teens most in need of counseling, abortion services, and/or prenatal services. Their responses, obtained through lengthy interviews, enabled us to compare the views and experiences of service recipients with the views and beliefs of the service providers and policy makers. In each community 35 adolescents who bore a child in 1976 were interviewed—in Farmville they were mothers aged 17 and younger who could be reached for an interview; 5 teenagers had moved or refused to be interviewed. In Southern City the 35 were a representative sample chosen to match the Farmville group. Their responses about to whom they first talked, others with whom they talked, and the persons whom they were careful not to let know of their pregnancy are given. After presenting the views of these teenage mothers we will compare their views with those of each of the policy-making boards and service-providing groups in order to look for trends, common impressions, and contrasts among the providers and recipients.

Telling the Boyfriend

Teenagers interviewed in both communities indicated a variety of different persons contacted when they first realized they were pregnant. In both groups the person with whom the teenagers first talked was most frequently the boyfriend: 31 percent (see Figure 3.2) in Farmville and 40 percent in Southern City. In more than half a dozen of these cases, girls reported that their boyfriend was the first person to notice the pregnancy. One girl told the interviewer that her boyfriend said that her stomach was getting hard. A second said that her boyfriend was sick. Another said that her boyfriend had morning

FIGURE 3.2

Persons with Whom Teenagers Who Became Mothers in 1976 First Talked about Their Pregnancies, Farmville and Southern City

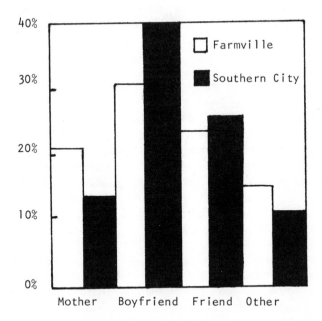

Note: N = 35 for each community.

Source: Constructed by the author.

sickness: "For two or three months he couldn't eat and he slept all the time." Yet another girl told the interviewer that her boyfriend suspected that she was pregnant because of the way she was acting.

Telling a Girl Friend

The next most frequently consulted person in both communities was a peer, usually female. Data indicated frequencies of 24 percent in Farmville and 26 percent in Southern City. Though peers generally tried to be helpful, the respondents' reporting of their reactions suggested that everyone saw the problem as belonging to the girl herself. The most usual response of a peer to being told her friend was pregnant was to ask what she intended to do about it. Some encouraged their friend not to have an abortion, to have the child and return to school. One teenager gave this report: "I told one of girl friends first. She didn't really say much. She just listened while I talked. She said, 'Go ahead and have it,' 'cause I was going to go ahead and have it anyway."

Considering these two groups of contacts together means that half the Farmville teenagers and two-thirds of the Southern City teenagers first talked either to their boyfriend or to a peer, usually a girl friend.

Telling Parents

Mothers of pregnant adolescents were consulted more frequently in Farmville than in Southern City: 21 percent of the teenagers talked to their mothers in Farmville; only 14 percent did in Southern City. Only one of these mothers was happy to know her daughter was pregnant; however, each of the girls indicated her mother's support. Support is more clearly evidenced in Farmville than in Southern City. One 17-year-old, Anna Swain, looked back on her pregnancy and commented on her mother's response:

Yeah, Mama was the first one to suspect I was pregnant. How did she know? I don't remember exactly what she said to me one day, something about "How come you ain't never asked for no Tampax?" I told her, "I guess I won't need them for nine months." After that we talked about my pregnancy and she asked me what I wanted to do about it. I told her I wasn't sure, but I knew that I was too young to have an abortion unless I had my parents' signature. She said that it was my decision what to do, but that she wasn't going to hell for nobody.

Anna's mother added her own perspective:

> Things are different now. In my day, if we got pregnant,
> we kept it a secret. I sure don't want my others daughters
> to have a baby before they get married. . . . When you have
> a baby, and you're not married, the baby's father takes you
> for granted. They think you're just gonna stay home and
> wait for him.

After the birth of her child, Anna continued to live at home. Her
mother is obviously very found of little Lorraine, and shares the responsibility of caring for her grandchild when Anna needs to go out.
At present Anna is living at home with both her parents, helping her
mother keep house. She has finished the eleventh grade and plans to
work toward her high school certificate. A previous pregnancy resulted in miscarriage when Anna was 16.

In Southern City mothers were less frequently the first to be
consulted, perhaps because of the greater availability of health care
alternatives, perhaps because of differences inherent in urban and
rural settings. Curiously, several mothers in Southern City seemed
to be waiting for their daughters to tell them the obvious. One mother
surprised her daughter by quietly reporting that she already knew the
girl was pregnant. She simply said, "Go to the doctor all the time."
Another mother said she had known because her daughter kept getting
dizzy.

Carrie Williams told the interviewer that her mother found out
before she did, because the doctor told Mrs. Williams, rather than
Carrie, after he had examined her. While Mrs. Williams was disappointed, she was also very relieved. Carrie had not menstruated for
two years, and thought she could not become pregnant. She had none
of the usual symptoms, and therefore did not suspect pregnancy.
Around the fifth month of her pregnancy, Carrie went to the doctor
because of stomach trouble. A cyst or stomach cancer was suspected.
However, after consulting with physicians from a nearby medical center, her doctor determined Carrie was pregnant. At that point abortion was no longer an alternative. Mrs. Williams made sure that
Carrie went faithfully to the doctor so that there would be no more
medical problems.

Teenagers in both communities avoided speaking directly with
their fathers, even after their pregnancies became known. No one
interviewed reported speaking to her father first. The more usual
pattern was for the girl's mother to tell her husband of the daughter's
pregnancy. Then, evidently, the daughter and father met in passing
and one mumbled something to the other. The father's disapproval
was clear in this repeated pattern of noncommunication. One Southern

City girl reported that her father merely said, "Good luck in havin' it." This pattern of reticence (and implied disapproval) was similar for both black and white fathers.

Between Parents and Daughters:
A Communications Gap

We also asked the teenage mothers to list all the other persons they talked with about their pregnancy (see Table 3.3). Ten percent in Farmville and 5 percent in Southern City never talked about the pregnancy with anyone aside from medical personnel. Although these figures are necessarily estimates, they do indicate clear trends for teens actually to talk with their boyfriends and girl friends, rather than with their parents or service agency personnel. By combining data from Figure 3.2 and Table 3.3, we find that half of the teens interviewed talked to their mothers. And eventually 20 percent of rural

TABLE 3.3

Other Persons with Whom Teenagers Who Became Mothers in 1976 Talked about Their Pregnancies, Farmville and Southern City, 1977 (percent)

Person	Farmville	Southern City
Husband	3	0
Boyfriend	61	43
Father	18	29
Mother	30	43
Minister	0	6
Family planning worker	9	17
Social worker	6	23
Guidance counselor	3	11
Other person	42	34
No one else	9	6

Note: N = 35 for Farmville and for Southern City.

Source: Compiled by the author.

teenage mothers and 30 percent of urban teenage mothers talked with their fathers. We cannot speak to the quality or satisfaction of these talks. What is a clear trend, however, is for little communication to occur between pregnant teenage daughters and their mothers, and even less between daughters and fathers. Again, this might not be a distressing situation if other satisfactory avenues were open and being used by the pregnant teen.

An emerging trend that we shall see throughout the data in this and the following chapters is for pregnant urban teenagers to have more options and to exercise them to get help. For example, while the figures are admittedly small, twice as many Southern City pregnant teenagers talked to a family planning worker and four times as many talked to a guidance counselor as did the teens in Farmville.

Figure 3.3 gives information on those people from whom pregnant teenagers at first felt it was important to conceal their pregnancy. The teenagers interviewed reported that they were very careful not to let their mothers know of their pregnancy. However, actual behavior of the adolescents of both cities varied from the stated norm. In Farmville further questioning of the teenagers indicated that the mother was the second most frequently consulted person. While the girls most often told their boyfriends of their pregnancy first, boyfriends were frequently less experienced and less knowledgeable about health care resources in the area and therefore were of little or no help in assisting the girl in dealing with her predicament. So, in spite of the anticipated repercussions of telling her mother, the girl knew that her mother would be able to provide helpful solutions. Since nearly 70 percent of the girls interviewed have lived in Farmville all their lives, it is logical to assume that their mothers would know of the services available. It is possible to conjecture that some mothers had used the same services themselves 15 to 18 years earlier, when their daughters were born.

Teens also reported that they were very careful not to let their fathers know of their pregnancy. In this instance their behavior was more in line with their reporting of the norm. None of the teens in Farmville reported speaking first with her father. This statement was supported by further questioning in informal conversation. Only two teenagers indicated that they had then told their fathers after telling either a boyfriend or their mothers. Patti Davis, one of these girls, had the following to say of her experience:

> I told my daddy after I told him [boyfriend] and my sister. He wanted me to have the baby, but he sure wasn't much help in suggesting what I should do with it. He didn't even know any places I could go while I was pregnant. I didn't bother my mama with my problem, as she has six

FIGURE 3.3

Persons Whom Teenagers Who Became Mothers in 1976 Did Not Immediately Tell of Their Pregnancy, Farmville and Southern City (number of times mentioned)

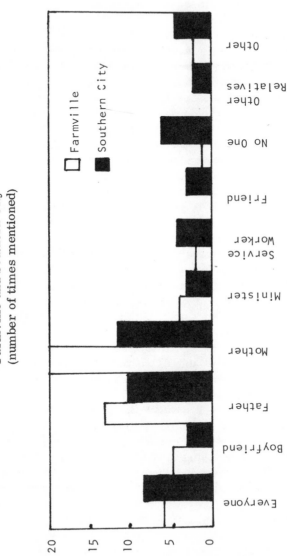

Source: Constructed by the author.

other children to take care of and no one to help her
with them.

Patti ultimately found her way to the Health Department, where she
continued her prenatal care until her child was born.

For various reasons, then, the teenagers who gave birth felt it
very important not to let their parents know of their pregnancy. Few
girls—15 percent in Farmville and 9 percent in Southern City—were
anxious that their boyfriends not find out; about 10 percent were very
careful not to let their minister find out; and 10 to 20 percent were
careful not to let anyone find out.

The clear trend, then, was for the teenagers who became pregnant and participated in this study to seek advice from their girl
friends and boyfriend, and to avoid seeking advice from, or even re-
vealing their situation to, their parents. If the girl's peers were well
informed, this occurrence might not in itself be bad; but as data in
later chapters show, the girl friends and boyfriend to whom pregnant
teens turn for advice are unlikely to be able to provide the counsel
needed. Parental advice is generally avoided, and few receive advice
from trained professionals. As a first step in exploring some of the
dynamics behind these behaviors of the girls who became pregnant in
the two communities, we will examine the views and thoughts of policy
makers, service providers, and the teenage and adult general public
on the questions of to whom teenage girls first talk and where they go
for help.

POLICY MAKERS' PERCEPTIONS

> I've seen a lot of them pregnant and have had their
> mothers and daddies talk to me.
> > A Farmville county commissioner

Views of the 13 elected county commissioners and city councilmen in the two communities varied between 7 who were aware that
peers are most often the initial persons to whom teens talk, and 2
commissioners who said they did not know. Of the first 7, 3 elabo-
rated no further than to say that peers or close friends are the most
likely first contact.

One top city administrator, who sat on the city council ex officio,
said teens go to friends first, then perhaps school personnel, then a
counselor, and finally to parents, but noted that they go to parents
too late. He added that in his experience they do not go to the city
agencies—a finding that the teens who delivered in 1976 tend to cor-
roborate. Another commented that pregnant adolescents first talk to

friends or some other trusted person, but that concern about a stigma attached to such a pregnancy prevents many from seeking help—much depends on the sexual partner. Our interviews with the teen mothers corroborated this statement.

One white county commissioner who operates a business commented that he had "not run into this" (learned to whom teens first talk). He added that if a pregnant teenager came to him for help, he would send her to the Health Department and would be especially concerned about her physical and mental well-being, that the first thing is to look after the health of mother and child. Although two commissioners thought pregnant adolescents always go to their parents, on balance the awareness level of the top elected and appointed officials in the two communities seemed relatively high.

Named Influentials

Of seven named influential community members interviewed, four cited peers and close friends as the first contact and two named parents or school personnel. The other, an automobile dealer, named the girl's sister as the most likely first contact.

Board of Mental Health and Health Department

Pregnant teens hide it as long as they can and are
not likely to say anything.
                    Mental health board member

When the responses of the mental health board members in the two communities are compared with those of the Health Department members, we find the first group is much more likely to view a peer, usually a close girl friend, as the pregnant teen's first contact. Health board members tended to name parents and school counselors.

Mental health board members in both communities tended to list several considerations, usually mentioning a peer as the first person with whom these young women are most likely to talk. One commented that it depends on the socioeconomic circumstances—middle-class girls go to the family doctor, minister, or school counselor, while lower-class girls go to the Department of Social Services or the Health Department. One mental health board member in her fifties, when asked in a home interview what school-age girls in her community do when they suspect pregnancy, turned to her 16-year-old daughter and asked, "What would you do if you thought you were pregnant?" The daughter replied without hesitation, "I'd go to Beaufort [a town nearby] and get an abortion."

The School Boards

> Seldom if ever a parent until it's too late.
>> A Southern City
>> school board member

The school board members in both communities seemed to have had prior thoughts about the problem of counseling help for teenagers who suspect pregnancy. The majority of the 18 board members interviewed mentioned peers and close friends as the first persons to whom these young women turn; 4 of them emphasized that teenagers tend to go to their parents "last."

Three comments typify the type of response school board members made. The first, the black member in her fifties quoted earlier, said, "The first thing most girls do when they find themselves pregnant is talk to their best friend, and next they seek advice from the male as to what they should do." The second board member, a white male life insurance salesman, commented, "A girl will discuss the situation with a close friend, maybe the school counselor, and possibly the boy, if known—she'd probably call a Southern City medical or abortion clinic listed in the yellow pages—when all else fails, she probably brings it to her mother." A third board member, black and in his forties, listed "(1) close friends, (2) someone outside the home who may have had experience, (3) a doctor who won't tell, or a sister, maybe, (4) seldom if ever a parent until it's too late."

SERVICE PROVIDERS' VIEW

Family Planning Clinic Staff

> Some never do [tell their parents].
>> A Southern City family
>> planning nurse

In both Southern City and Farmville the six key family planning staff persons in the Health Departments were interviewed at length. Without exception all viewed the parents as the last persons the teenager would tell. One family planning nurse practitioner commented, "Some never do." A family planning registered nurse in Southern City commented that sometimes teenagers in her clinic would talk to a favorite relative or to a close friend of their mother's in order to "get a feel for how Mom will take it."

Jessica Dare first told her boyfriend of her pregnancy, but then told her aunt before telling any other family members. The aunt lived in Baltimore but was visiting Jessica's mother. Her Aunt Rita advised Jessica to talk the situation over with her boyfriend and then suggested that she tell her mother. In fact, the aunt herself told Jessica's mother. According to Jessica, "She kind of helped me out a lot."

The family planning workers stated in every interview that peers—girl friends—are the first persons with whom their teenage clients talk. One Farmville staff member said, "We've had a lot call or get a friend to call about the pregnancy test, or if they call themselves, they say, 'I don't want my parents to know.'" Two workers felt there is a clear tendency to deny the pregnancy until it is obvious, thereby delaying talking to a friend—who, the staff member added, usually has "no factual information or knowledge."

One Southern City teen did not acknowledge that she was pregnant. Though she missed a period and had dizzy spells, she told no one that she thought she might be pregnant. "My mother found out when I was about five months," said Kristi. "I didn't tell her or nothing. She just figured it out." When asked to comment on her mother's reaction, Kristi said, "She told me to be calm and so forth, that it would soon be over with. I was too far along for an abortion."

Kristi started prenatal care in her fifth month of pregnancy, and her record indicates that she made only four prenatal visits. Her son was adopted by another black family. The adoption (the only one among the 70 teenage mothers interviewed), Kristi says now, was probably the right thing to do. At the time she was only 15, and her parents felt quite strongly that adoption was the best alternative. When asked her reasons for deciding to have her baby adopted, Kristi replied, "My parents told me to give up the baby for adoption." She still thinks about her son quite often, and told the interviewer that when he is 18, he will be able to find out who his real mother is. Kristi also said that she wished birth control and sex education were more available to young people.

The consensus among the family planning staff in Southern City is that the general sequence is first to tell a friend, second to talk with someone at school (such as a physical education teacher), next to seek help from the local Health Department, and finally to talk to a parent. The Farmville Health Department staff agreed, but added that the second most frequently talked-to person is the boyfriend, so the sequence would normally be girl friend, then boyfriend, then Health Department. Significantly, Farmville family planning staff members did not mention school counselors or physical education teachers among the initial persons with whom teens talk. This impression will be borne out later in our discussion of sex education practices and attitudes in these two communities.

A leading staff member in the Farmville Health Department, in pointing out the importance of friends as a major source of information for teens who suspect pregnancy, observed that often these friends refer the pregnant girl to a service agency. Referrals by friends had decreased lately, she said, then explained that such referrals follow a cycle of two or three years. A group of high school students who had made numerous referrals to their Health Department clinic had now gone to college.

The Private Physicians

> The girls run to men until they are pregnant, then run to me.
>
> A Farmville physician

Private medical doctors reported different patterns for the two communities. Half the private physicians interviewed in Farmville reported that teenage women who suspect pregnancy talk first with their girl friends, but half were of the opinion that the family doctor is the first person to whom the teens turn. One physician commented that girls go to the family doctor "especially here," saying that there was a "special relationship" with doctors in his community. Another physician commented that pregnant adolescents "usually go to their girl friends, and finally, and with frustration and hesitancy see their licensed medical doctor." Another physician said teens "don't go to the doctor or clinic first; they have a personal contact with someone."

If the Farmville physicians are oriented to private practice, the private physicians in Southern City, by contrast, are oriented to the Health Department. While most of the 14 private physicians mentioned girl friends as the first person with whom the teenagers talk, they were quick to add that girls then go to the local Health Department for help. One physician gave the following response:

> A pregnant girl's first reaction is fear—she'll do nothing —and then she'll come to the health department for a pregnancy test (low economic levels) or go to a private MD without her parents' knowledge. The result is referral of the upper socioeconomic level teenager for an abortion, with the lower socioeconomic girl coming to term, because there's no money for abortions.

The Pharmacists

> Pharmacists are a focal point for more than people give them credit for.
>
> A Farmville pharmacist

One pharmacist in each of the six drugstores in Farmville was interviewed. None reported that peers or close friends are the first person to whom teenage women turn. Two pharmacists felt that pharmacists are the first person with whom these young women talk. One druggist commented, "A certain percentage [he never specified] come to a pharmacist." Two felt teens go to their doctor first; one reported the Health Department as the first teen resource; one said Farmville teens "go out of town for a test." Of the five pharmacists in our Southern City sample, three reported peers as the first persons to whom young women who suspect pregnancy talk, one of them adding, "This leads to misinformation." One thought the parents were the most likely source of first help; one did not know.

Social Workers

> Most but not all teens wait several weeks or even months
> before informing anyone.
> > A Southern City social worker

Four of the nine social workers who deal with pregnant teens in Farmville had difficulty overcoming their institutional orientation, replying that teens suspecting pregnancy go either to the Health Department or to the social worker's office first. Four others had comments that give a feeling of how a social worker might view the situation. One responded, "(1) The first stage is panic and trying not to believe it; (2) Girls do not go first to the Department of Social Serviews; (3) The black poor go to a friendly neighborhood woman." The second social worker said, "The first contact is friends, another teen—girls don't seek professional help until the obvious signs force them—the schools bring teens to this agency." A third commented, "Girls tell their girl friends—they don't want to believe it or tell their parents—they tell others when they get sick or show." The fourth social worker stated, "They tell other girls first—they get information from friends, a few go to school or social services right away."

Southern City social workers report patterns similar to those reported by the Southern City private physicians. Among the sample of seven interviewed, the consensus was that girls first talk with peers, then go to the Health Department, and finally to the Department of Social Services. A 30-year-old social worker made the following comment: "Generally a family member is the first to be told—a mother, grandmother, an aunt, or other extended family member. It is usually the family member who makes the request for assistance. However, in cases where the teen is involved in a second pregnancy, she may request the services."

Kate Miller sought the advice of a family planning nurse who came regularly to check her sister's blood pressure. Though she did not ask directly for services, she hinted that she thought she might be pregnant for a second time. The nurse asked her how many periods she had missed, and then advised her to go to her family doctor. Kate reported that she had had two pregnancy tests. One was done at the public health clinic, the other by a private doctor. She chose to go to a private doctor for prenatal care because Dr. Reynolds had always been the family doctor and she was very fond of him. Her first child, a girl, had been born in July 1976. The second child, a son, was born 15 months later.

Mental Health Workers

Three service providers at the Farmville mental health center were identified as active in the area of teenage pregnancy. One of the three said "I don't know," one discussed the agency's crisis hotline, and the third made the following observation when asked to whom teenagers in the community first talk when they suspect pregnancy:

Blacks don't call in on the crisis line. For blacks, usually their mothers find out through missed periods and swelling stomach—usually they are six months pregnant by then. For whites it varies—last week a 15-year-old from a well-to-do family called. What can I do? Her parents were separated, her dad was away, and he was the only person she had confidence in.

The three similarly placed persons in the Southern City mental health center repeated the views obtained from Southern City physicians and social workers—a pattern of seeking out friends, then the Southern City Health Department; one of them commented, after mentioning friends, "but not the parents or other adults."

School Administrators

Not the high school counselor.
A Southern City school principal

We interviewed ten school administrators in each community. About half the Farmville administrators mentioned peers or close friends as the first persons with whom the young women would talk. One principal in his fifties went out of his way to say "not the high

school counselor." Another principal in his sixties added that teens
are "least likely to go to teachers." Two administrators said they
did not know. Two observed that the teenagers first talk with their
peers, and that there is "no common pattern after that." One administrator mentioned that what happens varies with class: blacks wait
until they are showing to discuss their pregnancy with anyone, but
whites come to see her more frequently and earlier. A younger principal, of a school covering kindergarten through grade 12, said, "I
believe a girl would first talk with the boy involved and together they
would decide who to go to for help. Those who have strong relations
with parents would go to them soon, but others might seek out another
person they can confide in."

Southern City principals had much more positive feelings about
the probability that teenage women suspecting pregnancy would go to
school counselors. Seven mentioned school counselors as the first
resource to whom teens would turn; only two mentioned peers and
friends as the first resource. One administrator responded that from
her observation teens "(1) try to keep to themselves, hoping it's not
true they're pregnant, (2) confide in their best friend or boyfriend
rather than a parent, (3) some confide in the school counselor; a few
may go to a doctor."

School Counselors

Four school counselors were interviewed in Farmville. None
of them thought teens would talk first with their peers. One mentioned
the counselors (school, presumably) as the first contact, and one mentioned the family doctor. One said the "response varies with socioeconomic level and social class. In general, they consult their family
physician or gynecologist, or go to the county health department or
social services." One high school guidance counselor declined to
answer the question because she had only recently arrived in the community.

Of the three counselors interviewed in Southern City, two named
peers, then a counselor, and one named the school nurse, then a
counselor as the first persons to whom teens suspecting pregnancy
talk.

Ministers

Teenagers are afraid the minister will tell their parents.
                                                    A Farmville minister

Responses of 20 ministers in Farmville and 7 ministers in Southern City are difficult to categorize. Most gave lengthy answers that were rather involved and analytical. One fundamentalist pastor said he was "not aware of a single instance of teenage pregnancy." A second, known for his campaign against pornography, commented, "I don't know. This apparently is not a large problem in our community. I visit the hospital frequently and have seldom met a girl of school age delivering a child—your experience may be different."

However, 14 of the Farmville pastors and one of the Southern City pastors mentioned peers and close girl friends as the first persons to whom teens who suspect they are pregnant may talk. Ministers tended to see themselves as a major source of consultation.

In contrast, the teenagers indicated that ministers are relatively unimportant where the issue of early pregnancy is involved. Let us examine what they reported. In Farmville 33 of 35 teens interviewed indicated that they did not tell their minister of their pregnancy. Further, 29 of these teenagers indicated that they did not avoid letting the pastor know. The logical conclusion of these two pieces of data is that ministers were not important people in the teenagers' network.

In Southern City the data indicate almost the same situation. Here 34 of 36 teenagers interviewed indicated that they did not tell their pastor of their pregnancy. And 31 had no interest in making sure he did not know.

Therefore, though ministers in the two areas tended to see themselves as a major source of consultation by teens who suspect pregnancy, interviews of the teenagers themselves clearly indicated that the ministers' opinion does not apply to them.

When there is consultation, it is usually initiated by the parents rather than the teenager herself. One minister commented, "Parents come to ministers for help for them and the child—the father of a daughter needs the most help." One Protestant minister in Farmville commented that the "minister may be last—if the minister is moralistic. Usually the mother would come to the minister and bring the child." He added parenthetically that when he had been a counselor, he had a "great deal more advice to give than now as a minister."

The teenage father was not a focus of our study, and was seldom mentioned by those interviewed. However, one minister commented that while the pastor might be the last person to whome a teenage girl would come, the boy might come. He added that when teenagers come, boys or girls, they are afraid of "rebuke."

"Teenagers are afraid the minister will tell their parents," said another Protestant minister in Farmville. Yet another Protestant minister saw the pregnant teen first going to her boyfriend, "not peers or parents," then experiencing a lot of denial in her own mind, then going to the doctor, who informs the parents, who in turn inform the minister. A rural Protestant minister believed teens do come to the minister first because they "trust the confidentiality," adding that "children anticipate their parents will be outraged, and lose control over themselves." One clergyman reflected on the helplessness of many teens: "Most teenagers go to friends with experience; they want to abort—counselors and parents don't find out till the fourth or fifth month." The few ministers interviewed in Southern City saw teen-agers going first to their ministers and their mothers. One added, after saying that teens first tell the minister, teacher, or parents, "Recently the trend, in my situation, is often for the girl to seek abor-tion, keeping it as quiet as possible."

The General Public

> She thinks about knocking it up herself.
>   A 20-year-old black mother

We will examine responses first from Farmville, then from Southern City, moving from younger to older respondents' comments. One striking aspect of early pregnancy behavior as perceived by resi-dents of Farmville is that among blacks, illegal abortion is still a serious consideration, apparently because of the costs of a legal abor-tion. A 20-year-old black mother who is separated and earns about $5,000 a year working in a local store said:

> When a girl thinks she is pregnant, she goes to the doctor
> to make sure, then maybe she'll tell her best friend about
> it. First she thinks of abortion, then she thinks about
> knocking it up herself. If that don't work, she tells her
> mother and she makes arrangements for her to have an
> abortion.

The respondent then named three illegal abortionists in Farmville, all of them female, to whom local black girls turn. A 25-year-old married black mother of three children who has had training in textile work, but who is not currently working, said:

> I think some school-age girls in this county try to do away
> with their babies when they suspect that they are pregnant.
> They usually talk to other girls of their age that know about
> such things. Some may even go to other women that are
> older and know how to knock a baby up. A few go to the
> health clinic for help.

The father of two boys, a white store manager earning a high salary, commented:

> Girls talk to their close friends first, asking for advice
> because they know the parents will be furious. They
> turn to an out-of-town doctor for help because if they go
> to a doctor in the same town or family doctor, he will in-
> form the parents as soon as the girl's back is turned.

A 41-year-old white housewife with one child and a 44-year-old white working mother with one child see teenage behavior, especially black teenage behavior, differently. In the view of the housewife:

> Usually the girl will tell the male involved that she sus-
> pects pregnancy. When she gets no assurance from him,
> she will turn to her parents as a last resort. In my opin-
> ion the females of the minority feel no guilt or remorse
> concerning their problem. Minority females have a ten-
> dency to disallow abortions, unlike their counterparts.

The working mother observed:

> White girls go to the gynecologist or Farmville Hospital
> for pregnancy tests. Some may go to a family doctor or
> the public health service. They go to Beaufort for abor-
> tions. Black girls probably go to their family doctor or
> (I've heard this) to Dr. Rathkin for pregnancy tests.
> Some do go to the public health service. Most black
> girls do not have abortions.

Two persons in their forties mentioned South Carolina. One said, "Tell their boyfriend and head for South Carolina." The second said, "Run away to Dillon, South Carolina, then talk to mother." South Carolina has long been the traditional destination of elopers from North Carolina who think that it is easier and quicker to get married in Dillon or one of the other border towns—a belief that no longer holds as much truth as it once did.

A retired public utility employee in her seventies reflected concern about responsibilities and obligations of individuals:

> They talk to all their friends instead of going first to their
> parents or guardian—this to me is pathetic, because our
> parents who love us or our guardian who is responsible for
> us should be the first to know.

Responses in Southern City, with the exception of no mention of illegal abortion, were similar to those in Farmville. A 24-year-old unmarried woman working in a research lab in a nearby university put it simply: "A girl considers abortion, running away, suicide." A 24-year-old unmarried male meat cutter in a supermarket commented:

> The pregnant girl, a few months along, probably confides in a friend who can offer very little information and consolation. Afraid to face irate parents or people of authority who could offer sound alternatives, she waits till she is discovered. Then she has to bear the responsibility of an illegitimate child.

Markedly different levels of sophistication show up when one compares the answers of urban and rural teenagers in the general public sample who chose to complete the questionnaire sent to them. Of the eight Farmville teenagers, six knew of no agencies or persons to whom teens who suspect they may be pregnant can turn, though two of them mentioned "mother and daddy" and "preacher." Two Farmville teens mentioned the Health Department as a place to obtain tests and counseling. In contrast, of the 13 Southern City teenagers who responded, 10 knew of local clinics and doctors to whom teens could turn.

Overall, the level of information available among Southern City teenage respondents was impressively greater than among the rural adolescents. The Southern City group is oriented to clinics, Health Departments, family physicians, and crisis hotlines. The Farmville group is oriented to "mother and daddy" and the preacher. Both groups are very clear in their impression that the first person to whom a teen talks when she suspects she may be pregnant is a close girl friend. Parents are not thought of by either group as the first source for help. As one Southern City teenage male put it, the reaction is "panic, then they talk to girl friends, boyfriends, or the boy they have had relations with. Only as a last resort do they tell the parents, even if they have a good relationship." One 14-year-old Southern City girl expressed a position encountered over and over by family planning service workers in clinics, in terms of the probability of even encountering the problem of whom to talk to: "I don't really know, since all my friends aren't the kind, I think, to be pregnant."

SUMMARY

To whom, then, do teenage women in these two communities first talk when they suspect pregnancy? There seemed to be a consensus among all groups in our study that teenagers talk to their closest friends first and to their parents last. In between close friends or the boyfriend and the parents, there seemed to be no clear pattern. Most respondents apparently thought that the most critical element in the choice of a person to talk with beyond a peer is a relationship of trust. Sometimes this trust was accorded to the Health Department, sometimes to private physicians, sometimes to relatives or to other friends. There seemed to be no established pattern at all in Farmville. To the extent that there was an established pattern in Southern City, it was for teenagers who suspected they were pregnant to turn to the Health Department or to local abortion clinics.

The significant point for our research into the management of adolescent fertility in these two communities is that there were no clearly established patterns of service awareness among, or of service use by, teenagers in either community. A powerful need for anonymity in dealing with the problem of a suspected or confirmed teenage pregnancy loomed large especially in Farmville. Both the teenagers and the adult community sensed that anonymity and confidentiality were crucial, but apparently lacking. Teenagers in the two communities who suspected they might be pregnant faced a difficult situation: Peers were their prime source of help, but peers are, from our point of view, ill-prepared to offer the help needed. Most teenagers considered parents to be their last resort. They were unaware of agencies and sources of counseling available in the community, and feared that confidentiality could not be guaranteed even by an agency or professional counselor.

A number of service providers pointed out race-based differences between black and white pregnant teenagers. While we have focused our emphasis on teenage pregnancy as an adolescent rather than a racial problem, we did note two singular differences between blacks and whites: attitudes toward marriage and education. These differences are discussed in Appendix D.

4

TEEN ACCESS TO PREGNANCY TESTS AND PROFESSIONAL COUNSELING

PREGNANCY TESTS IN FARMVILLE AND SOUTHERN CITY

> [The Health Department has to] discourage willy-nilly pregnancy tests.
>
> A Farmville
> family planning physician

One of the measures of community attitudes toward sexuality is the degree to which pregnancy tests are made available or unavailable, easy or hard to get. We believe that access to pregnancy tests is an important indicator of a community's commitment to helping residents manage their fertility successfully.

During 1976 the Southern City Health Department gave 4,270 pregnancy tests. In that same year the Farmville Health Department, according to their reports submitted to the statewide family planning information system, gave 20 pregnancy tests. On the basis of Southern City data for the first six months of 1977 (see Figure 4.1), we can estimate that for 1976 a reasonably accurate figure would be 244 pregnancy tests to persons aged 13 to 16 and 848 tests to persons aged 17 to 19, or a total of 1,092 tests obtained by teenagers at the Health Department lab. It is not possible to know how many of the 20 pregnancy tests reported by the Farmville Health Department were given to teenagers, and whether they were positive or negative. Of the 4,270 tests given by the Southern City Health Department, 47 percent (1,995) were positive and 53 percent (2,275) were negative. We might make a crude guess by assuming that the ratio of positives to negatives is approximately the same for teenagers as for the total population: then more than 100 pregnancy tests given to teenagers aged 13 to 16

FIGURE 4.1

Percentage Distribution, by Age, of Pregnancy Tests Performed at
Southern City Health Department, January-June 1977

Ages 13-16

6% (122)   100%

Ages 17-19

22% (424)   100%

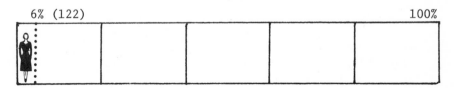

Ages 20 and over

72% (1,407)   100%

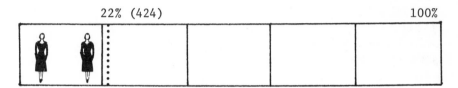

Note: N = 1,953.

Source: Constructed by the author.

were positive and 400 to teenagers aged 17 to 19 were positive. We
will clarify the pregnancy test management decisions made and en-
dorsed in the two communities below. Some additional perspective
can be gained on these figures by examining the views of various
groups in these two communities.

Table 4.1 gives an aggregated overview of the beliefs of policy
makers, service providers, and the general public in the two communities about where teenagers go to get pregnancy tests. All groups

TABLE 4.1

Where Teenagers Seek Pregnancy Tests: Views of Policy Makers,
Service Providers, and General Public, Farmville and Southern
City, 1977
(percent)

	Policy Makers		Service Providers		General Public	
	F	SC	F	SC	F	SC
Medical doctor	49	28	48	19	44	30
Public Health Department	37	46	40	43	38	41
Hospital	4	10	3	20	6	17
Outside the county	5	0	6	0	5	0
Private clinics	0	4	0	15	3	6
Department of Social Services	0	0	0	0	0	0
Charities	0	1	0	1	0	2
No service available	0	0	0	0	2	0
Other	5	11	3	2	2	4
Total	100	100	100	100	100	100
Number	63	62	54	55	313	309

Note: F = Farmville; SC = Southern City.

Source: Compiled by the author.

in both communities believed that about 40 percent of the time, teens
suspecting pregnancy go to the local Health Department. Southern
City residents believed that this occurred about 5 percent more frequently in their community than did persons living in Farmville.
Conversely, Farmville residents believed teens suspecting pregnancy
go to a private physician about twice as frequently as did Southern
City residents. Physicians in Farmville believed the community was
highly oriented to private physicians, more so than Southern City,
and the trends represented in Table 4.1 seem to confirm this belief.
The local Health Department and private physicians were clearly the
two places where most respondents felt that teens who suspect pregnancy go for tests.

Southern City adults and teenagers believed there were several
sources of services within the community, and thus no necessity to
go elsewhere. Farmville adults and teenagers believed there were

fewer sources for pregnancy tests available, and saw some pattern of going outside the community—possibly for anonymity, possibly simply to obtain services.

Teenage Mothers' Experiences

In Southern City, 97 percent of the teenage mothers had pregnancy tests: 18 at the public health clinic, 13 at the hospital, and 3 at the office of a private physician. Nearly 40 percent of this group went for a test as soon as they suspected pregnancy.

In Farmville only slightly over 70 percent of the teen mothers interviewed had had pregnancy tests. Of these, 15 had the test done at the public health clinic, 8 reported going to a private doctor, and 3 went to the hospital for the test. Apparently the local hospital had set up an effective barrier to testing teenagers by accepting referrals only.

More Farmville teenagers waited for one or two months before having a pregnancy test (51.4 percent); 22 percent of the girls had pregnancy tests done as soon as they suspected; 17 percent of the sample interviewed reported they had never had a pregnancy test. This fact may be due either to the difficulty of obtaining a pregnancy test in Farmville or to the fact that girls in Farmville more often deny their pregnancy until it is so apparent that no test is needed for confirmation.

Obtaining a Pregnancy Test

Southern City

For the Southern City teenager who suspects pregnancy there are, in addition to going outside the community (which is seldom mentioned), four routes to a pregnancy test.

Route 1: Public Health Department. A girl can take an early morning urine sample to the Health Department laboratory any time after 8:00 A.M. any weekday. The fee is $3, and results are available in three hours. Age is not a factor.

Route 2: Hospitals. Urine tests are available in the Outpatient Department of several of the city's eight hospitals. The fee is $8, and results are available later that day.

Route 3: Local Abortion Clinics. Pregnancy tests may be obtained at local abortion clinics. Costs and turnaround time vary.

Route 4: Private Physician. The most expensive route for a pregnancy test is via a private physician. The typical charge for the test
alone is $12. Turnaround time varies with the physician.

One member of the Health Department family planning staff estimated that 80 percent of teenagers wanting a pregnancy test go to the
Health Department. Of the 14 private physicians interviewed in
Southern City, 12 named both the Health Department and the private
physician as the main sources of pregnancy tests in the community.
One doctor named only the Health Department. A white, 36-year-old
physician said she did not know where teenagers could get pregnancy
tests in Southern City.

Farmville

For the Farmville teenager who suspects pregnancy there are,
in addition to going outside the community (which is frequently mentioned by respondents), two routes to a pregnancy test.

Route 1: Public Health Department. A teenager who calls or visits
the Health Department is asked the following questions:

1. Why do you want the pregnancy test? (The girl must have
missed at least two periods.)
2. How old are you? (If she is under 18, the girl must have
her mother's signature.)
3. Who is your family physician? (If the girl names a family
physician, she is referred to her own doctor unless she is already a
registered family planning patient at the Health Department or insists
she wants an abortion.)

If a prospective patient has missed two periods and is already
registered at the family planning clinic or wants an abortion, she is
eligible to continue pursuing a pregnancy test by completing the following procedures.
The patient is given an appointment for the family planning clinic,
held each Monday at the Health Department between 9:00 A.M. and
4:00 P.M. The appointment is given on the condition that the girl
makes and keeps a prior appoint at the Department of Social Services,
accompanied by her mother with proof of income for certification of
eligibility for Medicaid or for Title 20. (Actually the Health Department will allow a girl to complete her family planning clinic appointment whether or not she is successful in obtaining certification at the
Department of Social Services, but the prospective patient is not told
this.)

FIGURE 4.2

Steps in Obtaining a Pregnancy Test at Farmville and Southern City
Health Departments

```
┌─────────────────────────────────────────────────────────────────────┐
│                           FARMVILLE                                   │
│                                                                       │
│  Call or visit Health Department                                      │
│         │                                                             │
│         ▼                                                             │
│  Answer questions abour age, family  ──►  If girl has a family doctor │
│  doctor, missed periods                   or has missed only one pe-  │
│                                           riod, no appointment is     │
│         │                                 given                       │
│         ▼                                                             │
│  If girl has no family doctor and has                                 │
│  missed two periods, appointment is                                   │
│  given            │                                                   │
│                   ▼                                                   │
│  Visit Department of Social Services ──►  If ineligible, girl may de- │
│  with mother; give proof of income;      cide not to keep appoint-   │
│  determine Medicaid or Title 20          ment                        │
│  eligibility                                                          │
│         │                                                             │
│         ▼                                                             │
│  If declared eligible, girl keeps clinic                              │
│  appointment (if under 18, girl's mother                              │
│  must sign consent); girl registers as                                │
│  regular family planning patient                                      │
│         │                                                             │
│         ▼                                                             │
│  Physician examines girl bimanually; ──►  If bimanual examination    │
│  if pregnancy status is unclear, preg-   gives clear signs of preg-  │
│  nancy test is authorized                nancy, no test is authorized│
│         │                                                             │
│         ▼                                                             │
│  Pregnancy test is performed free                                     │
└─────────────────────────────────────────────────────────────────────┘
```

```
┌─────────────────────────────────────────────────────────────────────┐
│                        SOUTHERN CITY                                  │
│                                                                       │
│  Present urine sample to laboratory at 8:00 A.M.; pay $3; leave phone │
│  number                         │                                     │
│                                 ▼                                     │
│  Call for results at 11:00 A.M. or receive call if phone number was   │
│  left                                                                 │
└─────────────────────────────────────────────────────────────────────┘
```

Source: Constructed by the author.

The next step is for the teenager to keep her Monday appointment at the family planning clinic. The teenager who seeks a pregnancy test receives a bimanual examination for pregnancy by the family planning physician, who may authorize a pregnancy test if there is evidence of pregnancy—and then only when the girl insists that she wishes an abortion. If a girl wants to keep her child, a test is not authorized. When it is properly authorized, there is no charge for the pregnancy test. For a comparison of obtaining a pregnancy test through public health facilities in the two study communities, see Figure 4.2.

Route 2: Private Physicians. Leading obstetrician-gynecologists offer a Latex agglutination test while the patient waits during office hours, or one may bring a urine sample to the doctor's office by 9:00 A.M., with the results available at noon. Cost for this test is $5. Most private physicians will perform the test or give the patient a lab slip authorizing the hosptial to perform a test. (No self-referred outpatient service for pregnancy tests is allowed at Farmville Hospital.)

Statistics on pregnancy tests for the teenagers we interviewed who delivered a child in 1976 in Southern City and Farmville appear in Figure 4.3: 46 percent (16) reported they received their pregnancy tests at the public health clinic in Farmville. Since the Farmville Health Department had reported giving only 20 tests in 1976, it seems likely that it underreported the number of pregnancy tests they performed that year. In any case, about half the respondents in both communities reported having obtained a pregnancy test at their local Health Department. Teenagers in Southern City were four times as likely as those in Farmville to have obtained a pregnancy test at a local hospital. Farmville teenagers were about three times as likely to have gone to a private physician, and six times as likely never to have obtained a pregnancy test at all.

We set out to determine the number of pregnancy tests obtained by teenagers in both communities. We found that this kind of data is virtually impossible to obtain, if for no other reason than the fact that most physicians in these two communities do not aggregate such data by age or residence. For example, the obstetrical practice of Farmville physicians was estimated to be about 40 percent out-of-community persons. It seems reasonable to believe that most family practitioners in both communities either will perform pregnancy tests for patients or will refer them to the local hospital or Health Department. How many tests are obtained through all service givers in both communities cannot be determined.

How do the approaches of the physicians who make the policy decisions about pregnancy tests in the two communities differ? The head of the Health Department in Southern City took the position that

FIGURE 4.3

Places Where Pregnancy Tests Were Obtained by Teenagers Who
Gave Birth in 1976, Farmville and Southern City

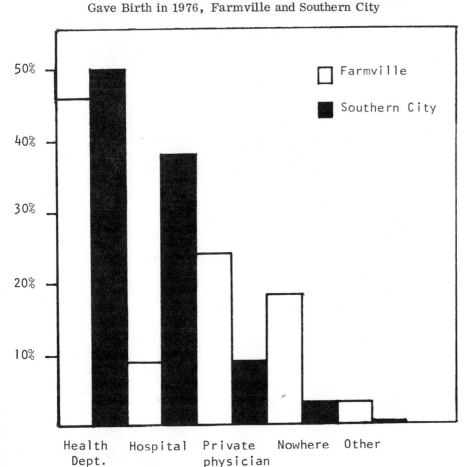

Source: Constructed by the author.

providing pregnancy tests and services for persons of all ages is a
necessary and desirable public service. He calculated that the test
material costs $1.25 and lab technician and secretarial costs amount
to $1.75; hence a cost of $3.00 to the patient. If a person cannot pay
the $3.00 fee, she can get the health educator at the family planning
clinic to authorize a free test.

The physician in charge of pregnancy test policy at the Farmville Health Department stated his philosophy as follows:

There must be limits. The pregnancy test should only be
performed for women who need it for some reason—abor-

FIGURE 4.4

Pregnancy Test Behavior of Teenage Mothers, Farmville and
Southern City, 1976

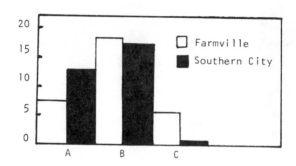

Statement: I went for a pregnancy test:

Answers: A -- immediately after I suspected I was pregnant.

            B -- one or two months after I suspected I was pregnant.

            C -- I never had a pregnancy test.

Note: N = 34 in Farmville; N = 33 in Southern City.

Source: Constructed by the author.

tion or contraceptive needs. Pregnancy tests cost $1.25
for supplies. . . . The pelvic or abdominal examination
before a pregnancy test serves a dual purpose: (1) to
discourage willy-nilly pregnancy tests and (2) to determine how fast we need to act.

The intake worker we interviewed agreed, adding, "We get a lot of
these little girls coming in wanting pregnancy tests. We couldn't keep
enough pregnancy test material on hand if we just served anybody who
walks in. We get so many calls . . . just curious people." One member of the professional staff at the Farmville Health Department cap-
sulized the department's position by saying, "Dr. Hyde is not too hip
on those pregnancy tests."

Olive Rogers discussed her own situation at length with the interviewer. She was 16 at the time of her first pregnancy. Though

young, and then unmarried, she was eager to have a child and recalled
feeling very relaxed about the pregnancy. She began telling people
she was pregnant even before she had a pregnancy test, and she started
a savings account for her baby. To obtain a pregnancy test, Olive had
to go to two different doctors. "Yep, the first doctor wouldn't give
me a pregnancy test. He wouldn't believe I was pregnant. He said I
was just stirring up trouble for my mom."

The physician referred Olive to the local mental health clinic.
Under their auspices Olive eventually received a pregnancy test as
part of a physical examination. "I guess they did a pregnancy test,"
Olive remarked, "because eight days later they told me I was pregnant. I already knew I was pregnant. I told them I was three months
pregnant so they put down three months. I don't know if they knew
other than what I told them."

While Olive's situation is admittedly unusual, the fact that it
happened at all is a strong suggestion that pregnancy tests are not
available for the asking in Farmville.

Pregnancy testing behavior of teenagers in the two communities
appears in Figure 4.4, which shows a larger proportion of Southern
City teenagers obtaining pregnancy tests immediately after suspecting
pregnancy, about an equal number obtaining pregnancy tests one to
two months after suspecting pregnancy, and a six times greater frequency of never obtaining a pregnancy test in Farmville. Policies on
pregnancy tests in the two communities, especially at the Health Departments, are indicative of different attitudes and practices regarding abortion, contraception, and sex education.

SOURCES OF COUNSELING HELP FOR
ADOLESCENTS WHO SUSPECT PREGNANCY

The physician who heads the Farmville Health Department family planning clinic said he prefers to do a manual examination for
pregnancy because time is of the essence. Teenagers, like all women,
are subject to the intense time-bound decision-making situation of
identifying the pregnancy and deciding to carry it to term or seeking
abortion.

Table 4.2 gives the views of policy makers, service providers,
and the general public on sources of counseling help. Clearly, Farmville policy makers and service providers felt there was counseling
help available to pregnant teens. The general public who responded
in Farmville felt differently: nearly 20 percent said flatly that there
were no sources of counseling help available, either individuals or
agencies, for pregnant Farmville teenagers. In contrast, virtually
all respondents in Southern City felt some counseling help was avail-

TABLE 4.2

Sources of Counseling Help for School-Age Young Women: Policy
Makers, Service Providers, and General Public, Farmville and
Southern City, 1977
(percent)

	Policy Makers		Service Providers		General Public	
	F	SC	F	SC	F	SC
None available	3	1	1	0	19	1
Public Health Department	15	25	21	27	22	22
Department of Social Services	13	15	18	15	17	13
Department of Mental Health	16	8	17	9	14	5
Churches	16	7	6	7	13	9
Schools	21	14	10	14	6	8
Private doctor	12	4	17	5	3	3
Hotline	0	3	0	1	0	8
Hospital	0	1	0	3	0	2
Charity	0	8	0	7	0	15
Clinic	0	1	0	8	0	7
Parents	0	0	0	0	0	0
Other	4	13	10	4	6	7
Total	100	100	100	100	100	100
Number	63	62	54	55	313	309

Note: F = Farmville; SC = Southern City.

Source: Compiled by the author.

able. This difference in perceptions between the general publics in
the two communities is reflected throughout their responses on availability of counseling help for pregnant teenagers in their communities.

In Farmville policy makers, service providers, and the general
public all agreed among themselves that the Health Department was
the prime source of counseling for teens who suspect pregnancy. Social services and the Department of Mental Health were the second
and third most often named sources. All three groups saw these
three agencies as available between 13 and 22 percent of the time.
Churches and schools were mentioned only infrequently. Surprisingly,
private physicians were believed to be a counseling source relatively

infrequently by policy makers and service providers, and by not more than 3 percent of the general public.

Southern City views showed the trend toward wide recognition of the Public Health Department. Policy makers, service providers, and the general public agreed that the Health Department was the most heavily used counseling source. The three groups viewed social services as about half as frequent a source of counseling. All three saw the Mental Health Department as about half again as frequent a source. As in Farmville, churches were consistently seen as a minor source (between 7 and 9 percent), as were schools (between 8 and 14 percent). The three groups considered the private doctor, the hotline, and the hospital insignificant sources of counseling help. The private clinics were seen as a more important source than any of the last three.

The 13 teenage respondents from the general public sample held clearly differing perceptions of the sources of counseling help in their two communities. Southern City teenagers were much more oriented to the Health Department as a counseling source—they named it twice as often as did teens in Farmville.

Comparisons between the Two Communities

What comparisons can be drawn between the two communities? The Health Department was the main source mentioned in both communities, significantly more so in Southern City. In both communities the Social Services Department was mentioned as a counseling source about half as often as the Health Department, the mental health facility about half again as often. The adult general public in both communities saw the schools as less frequently of help than did policy makers and service providers.

Private physicians were mentioned strikingly infrequently in both communities. In Farmville policy makers, service providers, and the general public mentioned private physicians between 3 and 17 percent of the time. In Southern City private physicians were mentioned 4, 5, and 3 percent of the time by policy makers, service providers, and the general public, respectively. Teens in the general public sample in both communities failed entirely to mention the private physician as a source of counseling help. Probably the largest single contrast between the two communities was that, as on other dimensions, there was a relatively wider selection of choices available in the urban setting.

The Mental Health Center

The county commissioners and city councilmen in Farmville emphasized a counseling service contribution by the county mental health center. Most of the time mental health was the first counseling source named. Several other groups of Farmville residents, including policy makers, reflected the belief that the mental health center was active in counseling teenagers with problem pregnancies. But the mental health center said it does virtually no counseling of teens who are pregnant or suspect pregnancy. The responses of local commissioners continued a trend of respondents in Southern City, naming a significantly larger variety of sources of help than their counterparts in Farmville. One commissioner said the Southern City Health Department did "nearly all" of the pregnancy counseling in the community. The influentials interviewed in Farmville frequently mentioned the school counselors as a major source of help. We were surprised when four of the seven members of the Southern City health board said they did not know what, if any, counseling sources were available in the community. Reflecting other respondents' similar beliefs, the majority of mental health board members in both communities believed their mental health center to be a source of counseling help.

The Schools

Farmville school board members had little hope of school counselors or other school personnel making much of a contribution to counseling assistance for Farmville teenagers who become pregnant. None of the seven members of the school board mentioned the schools as a useful source, and four never mentioned the schools. The first of the three who mentioned the schools said the school counselors "do not have the relationship with girls which would encourage this type of counseling. They are paper shufflers." The second school board member saw the counselor getting involved when the teenager is asked to discuss when to stop school. The third mentioned school counselors, then added immediately, "This community is pretty lacking in information. If counseling help is available, community teens probably are not aware of it." He added that a local physician had gone into the high school two years ago to give a lecture on birth control, and the parents "didn't like the frankness." Southern City school board members were equally pessimistic about schools helping in the counseling of pregnant teenagers. Among the school board members interviewed in Southern City, four said they knew of no counseling sources; four mentioned several sources, but never the schools; two mentioned school counselors.

Private Physicians and Pharmacists

Private physicians reflected pessimism about medical doctors as a source of counseling for pregnant teenagers. Among the nine medical doctors interviewed in Farmville, only one mentioned private

doctors as a source of counseling. One Farmville physician said "no
agency does" counseling. Three physicians said they did not know
whether or where counseling help might be offered in the community.
One mentioned the Children's Adoption Society in a nearby city as a
counseling source for placing adoptions. Another physician mentioned
the Young Mothers Association of Farmville, located in the obstetrics
ward at the hospital. Any decision to terminate a pregnancy would
likely have passed its time limit by the time the teenager came in contact with the Young Mothers Association. Southern City physicians
shared the Farmville physicians' views on private physicians as a
counseling source. Among the 14 participating Southern City physicians, 12 mentioned, among other sources, the Health Department;
one said "don't know"; and one said services are available but not
coordinated.

Pharmacists' responses in Farmville ranged widely. Two mentioned doctors and the health clinic, two mentioned only the Department of Social Services, one said only personal friends are available,
and one felt "no counseling is available." Southern City pharmacists'
responses also varied widely. One mentioned only Birth Choice (an
antiabortion counseling group), two mentioned the Health Department,
one mentioned guidance counselors in school, and one did not know.
The family physician across the street from his pharmacy was the
only source he knew of.

Social Services

> Teenagers make inappropriate plans.
>   A Farmville social worker

As might be expected, in both communities social workers, who
are closer to unintended pregnancies among teenagers, named several
sources. One trend among Farmville social workers was an emphasis
that the Health Department is not a satisfactory source of counseling
help. For example, one social worker commented, "I do not view
the Health Department as doing pregnancy counseling. The Health
Department pushes sterilization." A second social worker emphasized that social workers refer their clients to private medical doctors, saying they used to send them to the Health Department, but
the department sees patients only one day a week and only after two
missed periods. "That's late," the social worker added. "We can
get them to a private physician in hours." Another social worker
said the social worker assigned to the Health Department tells the
girls about birth control before pregnancy, but otherwise she did not
know where counseling help could be obtained.

What do social workers in Farmville see happening with teenage
girls' pregnancies? One commented that the sequence is for the teen-

ager to get pregnant and have the baby, then six months later to bring the baby to the Department of Social Services for foster care. "Teenagers," the social worker stated, "make inappropriate plans—that is, they neglect the child."

Southern City social workers named a variety of sources of counseling help. The single consistent source named by all but one social worker was the Health Department.

School Personnel

The school administrators in both communities, who, like social workers, are more familiar with teenage pregnancy, named a variety of sources for pregnancy counseling in their communities. Among the ten participating Farmville school administrators, five mentioned the Health Department, two said "no counseling is available in the community," and the others mentioned several sources. Half of the administrators said the schools in Farmville provide counseling help. Similarly, nearly half the Southern City school administrators thought the schools were providing counseling services, while half thought the schools provided none. School administrators, along with most other Southern City service providers, believed the Public Health Department was providing counseling services. Half the school counselors interviewed in Farmville felt the schools were providing counseling services to teens who become pregnant, but half thought the opposite. Among the three school counselors interviewed in Southern City, two felt the schools were providing counseling services; one viewed the school counselor's role as that of referring students to the public health nurses in the school system.

The information pattern that clearly distinguishes Southern City from Farmville is reflected in the responses of the 23 teenagers in the general public who participated in the sample. Over half of the teenagers in both communities either said they did not know of any, or that no counseling was available in their community. Of the Farmville teenagers who felt they did know a counseling source, one mentioned the church as the only source and the other listed four different sources, heading the list with his clergyman and guidance counselors at school. In contrast, of the 13 teenagers responding in Southern City, nearly half mentioned the Public Health Department, most of them believing it to be the only source of counseling help.

What Actually Occurs

In analyzing the responses of groups in the two communities, the clearest trend that emerges is a belief in Farmville that few sources of counseling are available, in contrast with a belief in Southern City that a variety of counseling resources are available to teenagers who suspect pregnancy. In Southern City the Health Department was consistently viewed as the prime source. The evidence we found in the two communities tends to confirm these beliefs.

Farmville

In Farmville the physician heading the family planning clinic named hospitals, school nurses, and health educators, but did not mention the Health Department clinic as a major source of counseling help. This impression was confirmed by one of the head nurses at the family planning clinic, who said the clinic has no formal program and that if a pregnant teenager wanted counseling in all aspects of the decision, the clinic staff would refer her to the Children's Adoption Society. The Children's Adoption Society, however, objective as it may be in its presentations, is nevertheless an adoption agency and is located an hour's drive from Farmville. The teenager who comes to the Health Department is asked, for example, "Do you want this baby?" Undoubtedly the nurses there do a good deal of informal counseling of pregnant teenagers. Nevertheless, it is clear both from the clinic head and from the staff nurses that they do not see themselves as a serious source of counseling help for teenagers who need to decide what to do about a problem pregnancy.

We have already seen the hurdles teenagers must overcome in order to get into the Farmville Health Department clinic for a pregnancy test. In essence, the Health Department staff members act on the teenager's decision, which is presumed to be made, to bear the child or to seek an abortion. As already described, teenagers who call the Health Department when they suspect pregnancy are told they are not eligible for help unless they have missed two periods and have a parent's signature along with Medicaid or Title 20 certification from the Department of Social Services. Surely there are some hardy souls who go to the Health Department without observing all the required procedures and get some advice from the staff, but these are probably occasional or rare instances. For the vast majority of teenagers in Farmville who seek advice on whether they are pregnant and what to do if they are, the Health Department is not a ready source of help.

The Department of Social Services in Farmville was viewed by several groups of participants in the study as a major source of counseling for pregnant teenagers in their community. The social workers estimated that they counseled 94 such young women during the 12 months prior to their being interviewed. This suggests a case load of nearly 100 teenagers in a year's time. Teenagers who present themselves to the Department of Social Services are sent to discuss their problem with the intake social worker, who works primarily with adoptions and maternity homes. From our interviews with the social work staff, it is clear that some of them discuss all the alternatives available to the teenager and help her make a decision, while some discuss only two or three of the four options (abortion, adoption, single parenthood, or married parenthood).

Another problem with the Department of Social Services is that it is set up to serve persons who qualify economically for receiving its services. For young women whose mothers are on the department's rolls, the possibility of going to see a social worker whom they have already met seems a logical step, although a relative usually makes the actual referral. But the young teenager who on her own seeks help from the social worker tends to be one who has already borne a child and is pregnant for a second time.

The first time a teenager gets pregnant, the reported pattern is for a relative to bring her to the Department of Social Services for help. It appears, then, that there is some use of the social workers, but seldom on a self-referral basis unless one pregnancy has already occurred, and usually not until the pregnancy is two or more months advanced. There are exceptions; the social workers report instances where the teenager refers herself, and gets assistance from the department in obtaining an abortion without her family having to know. These instances are clearly not the routine.

In short, while the Department of Social Services is a valuable community resource, it is regarded mainly as serving the low-income person. In the actual behavior patterns of Farmville teenagers, there appears to be only sporadic use of the social workers as sources of early counseling on the decision to seek pregnancy termination or enter into prenatal care.

The mental health program in Farmville was perceived by community policy makers and service providers as a significant source of counseling for teenage women who suspect a pregnancy. Is the mental health center a significant resource? Apparently not. If a teenager comes into the center for help, she must get a parent's consent before she can be seen. If she cannot or will not get parental consent, she is asked who else she is close to, such as a friend or minister. She is then asked to get her counseling from one of these persons. If the teenager calls in on the hotline, she can talk about the problem with the worker answering the telephone; but, as the mental health staff person said, "We do make referrals on the phone, but we don't do therapy on the phone." The three staff members at the mental health center who treat teenagers all said the center would provide the counseling if asked to do so (assuming parental consent is obtained). But few teenagers ask the mental health center for counseling assistance. The center staff estimated that five or six teenagers use the hotline each year for help with problem pregnancies. What specific advice was given is not known. The persons operating the hotline are not trained in dealing with problem pregnancies.

If teenagers in Farmville do not get significant amounts of counseling assistance from the Health Department or from the Department of Social Services, what other major sources might there be? The private physicians were the next most frequently thought-of counseling source, but only two of the nine physicians in Farmville named private physicians as a source of pregnancy counseling. It appears that private physicians, for the most part, do not see counseling pregnant teenagers as a priority aspect of their medical practice. They tend to think of the Department of Social Services, ministers, and the Health Department when asked who should provide counseling services to teenagers who suspect they are pregnant. As seen earlier, the perception that pregnancy counseling is not the job of the private physician is shared by the policy makers, service providers, and the general public, especially the teenagers, in Farmville.

If the physicians cannot or do not provide counseling on problem pregnancy, do school counselors? We interviewed four key school counselors believed by their principals and others to be involved in pregnancy counseling. The counselors said they believed the schools were providing counseling. However, of the four we interviewed, none had counseled teenage students about pregnancy within a year of the interview, although one had had contact with ten such women in the home-instruction program for teens whose pregnancies were advanced.

The final source we investigated within the service community was pharmacists, who might provide counseling for pregnant teenagers even though not formally trained for this task. None of the pharmacists interviewed, however, saw pharmacists as doing this kind of counseling, nor did any report they provided such counseling.

Ministers are frequently trained in counseling young persons. Of the 18 ministers interviewed, 30 percent felt the church was a significant source of counseling in Farmville for teenagers who become pregnant. We interviewed all the members of the Ministerial Association and a randomly selected group of 6 ministers who were not members (out of a total of about 56 ministers in the community). The number of teenagers with problem pregnancies counseled in the 12 months from June 1976 through May 1977 was not great: seven ministers counseled no teenagers with problem pregnancies, six counseled one each, two counseled five, one counseled six, and two counseled eight teenagers. The total number of teenagers counseled by 20 ministers in Farmville in 1976/77 was 38. More than half of the ministers would not discuss abortion as an option.

What, then, is actually happening in the provision of counseling services for teenagers who suspect or confirm a pregnancy in Farmville? A few are receiving help at the Department of Social Services, and a few are getting counseling from ministers. We accumulated little evidence that the Public Health Department, the Mental Health Department, the school, or private doctors provide counseling services to pregnant teenagers in Farmville. Although there may be more counseling actually being delivered than we were able to record, it is surprising to find the impression among respondents that community agencies and private physicians are providing counseling at a meaningful level.

Southern City

The Southern City experience is different. Clear impressions of a variety of sources of counseling for pregnant teens, focused primarily on the Health Department, are reflected from group to group in our study. The following places are additional counseling sources seen as available to Southern City teens that are presumed not to be available to Farmville teens:

Urban Information Center
Urban Social Ministries
Rape Crisis Center
Family Service/Travelers Aid
Inner City Satellite Center
Urban Opportunities Center
Local abortion and medical clinics
Positive Human Development Program
Salvation Army
Catholic Social Services
Four local college health services

We did not attempt to interview and collect data on the actual number of pregnancy counseling sessions held by each of the named places. The variety of counseling sources perceived by respondents as available is impressive. Since most of these counseling sources were named by service providers in a good position to know what resources are available and used, we presume that a teenager could at least get referral to professionally trained counselors in a number of the agencies and groups named.

There are, then, a number of places available to Southern City teenagers for at least a first contact that can result in actual counseling or in referral. When referral occurs, it is usually to the Health Department. A health educator hired by the department and trained in counseling pregnant teenagers said she counsels between 120 and 150 individuals each year. In addition to the health educator, there is a group of nurses trained in family planning who counsel teenagers visiting the family planning clinic. It is not possible to estimate the number of teenagers counseled by these nurses, inasmuch as this type of counseling is informal and varies from a very brief discussion to a lengthy interview and exploration with the girl about her feelings. It appears reasonable to believe that actual pregnancy counseling occurs not only at the Health Department but also at the Department of Social Services and mental health center, inasmuch as staffs from both of these places report that their centers provide counseling. The primary impression among Southern City school counselors was that while they do some pregnancy counseling, the usual procedure is to refer teens to the Health Department for professional counseling. Similarly, the private physicians in Southern City saw a pattern for pregnant teens to be referred by physicians to the Health Department for counseling.

Contrasts between the Two Communities

The most significant contrast between the responses of service providers in the two communities is that most service providers in Southern City knew of and mentioned the Public Health Department as the place to which they make referrals, then named several other sources of counseling, such as abortion clinics and the Children's Adoption Society. In sharp contrast, the Farmville service providers did not identify any single major referral agency, and exhibited no common knowledge of how or to whom teenagers in Farmville are referred. In short, there is a commonly known and used system of referrals to a central agency (the Health Department) in Southern City, but no pattern of referral to any agency or group in Farmville.

ESTIMATES OF EXTENT OF UNMET NEED

In Figure 4.5 and Table 4.3 we offer our analysis of the extent to which the estimated need for pregnancy tests and pregnancy counseling is being met in the two communities. Our figures are based on several assumptions and on incomplete data. We believe, however, that the results of our estimates are consistent with the estimates of types and amounts of need being met in the two communities.

Need for Pregnancy Test

The single most important assumption on which Table 4.3 and Figure 4.5 are based is the Alan Guttmacher Institute estimate that

TABLE 4.3

Family Planning Program Summary, Farmville, 1976

			Number of Patients				
	New	Continuing	Readmission	Transfer	Potential	Closed	Total
Total	262	349	55	1	0	264	931
Contraceptive services	261	349	55	1	0	3	669
Counseling	260	348	55	1	0	2	666
Treatment	1	9	0	0	0	0	10
Supply	253	332	55	1	0	2	643
Abortion referral	3	0	0	0	0	1	4
Sterilization referral	1	0	0	0	0	0	1
Infertility services	1	0	0	0	0	0	1
Other services	1	1	0	0	0	0	2
Counseling	0	0	0	0	0	0	0
Treatment	0	0	0	0	0	0	0
Babysitting	0	0	0	0	0	0	0
Transportation	0	0	0	0	0	0	0
Medical referral	1	1	0	0	0	0	2
Social referral	0	0	0	0	0	0	0
Mental health referral	0	0	0	0	0	0	0
Other	0	0	0	0	0	0	0
Medical services	262	344	55	1	0	6	668
Breast examination	259	336	55	1	0	3	654
Heart and lung examination	260	336	55	1	0	3	655
Pelvic examination	258	339	55	1	0	3	656
Pap smear	255	340	52	1	0	2	650
Gonorrhea test	256	340	54	1	0	4	655
Serology	259	336	55	1	0	3	654
Blood test	261	335	55	1	0	3	655
Pregnancy test	8	6	2	0	0	4	20
Urinalysis	262	334	55	1	0	3	655

Vaginal smear	0	3	0	0	0	0	3
Blood pressure	261	335	55	1	0	3	655
Other lab tests	261	335	55	1	0	3	655
Other medical examinations	261	335	55	1	0	3	655
Contraceptive method	253	338	50	1	0	6	648
Oral	235	314	48	1	0	0	598
IUD	12	16	1	0	0	0	29
Diaphragm	1	0	1	0	0	0	1
Foam, jelly	2	3	0	0	0	0	6
Rhythm	0	0	0	0	0	0	0
Condom	0	0	0	0	0	0	0
Injection	0	0	0	0	0	0	0
Sterilization	0	0	0	0	0	0	0
Withdrawal	0	0	0	0	0	0	0
Other	0	0	0	0	0	0	0
None	8	5	0	0	0	6	19

Medicaid-reimbursable visits	
Initial and annual medical	37
Medical with pelvic examination	2
Medical without pelvic examination	0
Title 20-reimbursable visits	
Initial and annual visits	158
Medical with pelvic examination	4
Medical without pelvic examination	2
Supplemental services reported	
Medical services	1,415
Supply visits	1,335
Outreach contacts	963
Lectures	0
Telephone contacts	3,620
Auxiliary services	0
Other	20

Source: North Carolina Division of Health, Department of Human Resources.

FIGURE 4.5

Estimated Number of Females Aged 13 to 18 in Need of Pregnancy
Tests and Number Receiving Tests through Public Health
Department, Farmville and Southern City, 1976

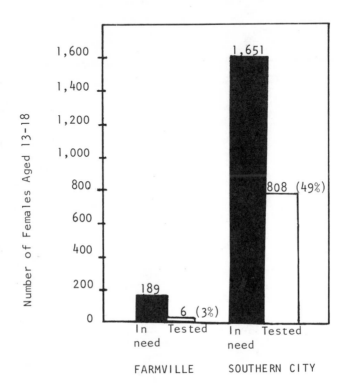

Source: Constructed by the author.

10 percent of U.S. females aged 15 to 19 become pregnant each year.
Using this percentage as a rough guide to the number of females aged
13 to 18 in both communities who are in need of a pregnancy test or
pregnancy counseling each year, we obtained the results shown above.

The Health Department in Farmville is meeting between 2 and
4 percent of the need for pregnancy tests (see Figure 4.5). It is known
that physicians, in their private offices and through use of the Farmville Hospital laboratory, provide an unknown additional number of
pregnancy tests for teenagers each year. In addition, the responses
from persons interviewed indicate that an unknown number of teenagers go to out-of-county hospitals and abortion clinics each year in
order to obtain pregnancy tests. In contrast, the Health Department

in Southern City meets approximately half of the identified need for pregnancy tests among females aged 13 to 18 each year. These proportions of need being met by the two Public Health Departments are consonant with the impressions of the policy makers, service providers, teenagers, and the general public in Southern City. (See Figure 4.5.)

On the basis of data obtained in our study, Farmville policy makers, service providers, teenagers, and the general public grossly overestimate the extent to which the Health Department is actually meeting the needs for pregnancy tests for teenagers. These data are straightforward and uncomplicated estimates of need. If the rate of approximately 50 percent positive results for all pregnancy tests conducted by the Health Department in Southern City is taken to mean that half the number in need are actually being reached through positive pregnancy identification, the effective percentage of need met by the Health Departments in both communities would be reduced by half. Or the proportion of need met could be recalculated on the assumption that fewer 13- and 14-year-olds become pregnant than 15- to 19-year-olds, which would reduce the percent getting pregnant each year to slightly less than 10 percent.

Need for Counseling

Using the same assumption that 10 percent of the teenagers become pregnant in each community each year, a rough idea of the need for pregnancy counseling can be obtained. In Table 4.4, 189 teenagers in Farmville are identified as in need of pregnancy counseling in 1976. It was possible to identify 110 who were reported to have been served by the service providers in our study at some point in their pregnancies. Our survey of ministers, the Health Department, and the Social Services Department was reasonably complete. Only those reporting that they counseled teenagers on all four alternatives (abortion, adoption, keeping the child with marriage, and keeping the child without marriage) are included in the table. Approximately 58 percent of the identified need for pregnancy counseling for teenagers in Farmville was met at some point during their pregnancy in 1976. It is impossible to offer a comparative estimate of the percentage of need met in Southern City during the same year, since we did not do 100 percent interviewing in Southern City because of its size.

Our data are necessarily rough estimates. There is nothing available to enable us to determine the quality of counseling or when counseling is sought in the two communities. We take these figures to be useful in indicating directions of need and of approximate proportions of need met and unmet. On the basis of these data we can

TABLE 4.4

Estimated Number of Young Women Aged 13 to 18 in Need of Pregnancy Counseling and Receiving Counseling
through Public Agencies and Ministers, Farmville and Southern City, 1976

	Farmville	Southern City
Number of teens		
White	1,394	12,252
Black	499	4,263
Total	1,893	16,515
Number needing pregnancy counseling	189	1,651
Number receiving counseling on all		
options (by source)		
Ministers	21	*
Health Department	8	*
Department of Social Services	81	*
Need met (percent)	58	Unknown

*Unable to estimate.

Note: Estimates are based on the Alan Guttmacher Institute (1976) estimate that 10 percent of U.S. females
aged 15 to 19 become pregnant each year.

Source: Compiled by the author.

say that the Public Health Department in Southern City does a better job of providing a significant proportion of the pregnancy tests needed by teenagers than does the Health Department in Farmville. It is not possible to estimate the extent to which both communities were meeting the need for pregnancy counseling for girls aged 13 to 18 in 1976 because of the very important factor of timing. Our interviews with the teenage mothers in these two communities revealed that they tended to seek counseling only after the pregnancy was toward the end of the first trimester, or past the time when an early abortion could be obtained.

FEELINGS IN THE TWO COMMUNITIES
ABOUT MEETING THESE NEEDS

One of our major research concerns was to test how people in all walks of life felt about the desirability of making the policies recommended by the American Public Health Association (APHA) the policies of their own community. To accomplish this, we asked persons throughout the two study communities how much they personally favored or opposed the APHA policies for their communities. To provide added perspective on the values held by the persons surveyed, we asked their counterparts at the state and national levels. (The methodologies and response rates were discussed in Chapter 2.) We turn now to a comparison of values held in these two communities by officials in their state government, and by similarly positioned persons at the national level. It will not be surprising that there is widespread support for stressing the need for early pregnancy tests and for discussing all alternatives with pregnant teenagers.

Figures 4.6 and 4.7 demonstrate a support for service programs to encourage teenage girls who believe they may be pregnant to get a pregnancy test as early as possible. Policy makers in both communities strongly supported early pregnancy testing for teenagers as a public policy. Service providers in both communities favored this idea to an even greater extent. Similarly, the general public in both communities strongly backed this approach to pregnancy management. The teenage mothers were less supportive. The reasons why teenage mothers appeared to be less supportive will be explored in our discussion of their life views, information levels, and the value influences acting upon them.

Strong support for a policy of stressing early pregnancy tests also existed among the North Carolina state judges and legislators. The national congressmen who responded were less supportive than North Carolina legislators. Human services administrators (HSAs) at both the state and national levels were practically unanimous in favoring early pregnancy tests for teenagers. (See Figure 4.8.)

FIGURE 4.6

Attitudes toward a Policy of Stressing Early Pregnancy Tests, Farmville, 1977

	Policy Makers (N = 63)	Service Providers (N = 54)	Adult General Public (N = 313)	Teenage Mothers (N = 35)
Favor strongly	0000000000 0000000000 0000000000 0000000000 0000000000 0000000000 00000000	0000000000 0000000000 0000000000 0000000000 0000000000 0000000000 0000000000 000	0000000000 0000000000 0000000000 0000000000 0000000000 0000000000 0000000000 000000000	0000000000 0000000000 0000000000 0000000000 0000000000 0000000000 0
Favor moderately	0000000000 0000000000 0	0000000000 000000	0000000000 000 000000000	0000000000 0000000000
Not sure	0000000000 0	000	000	0000000
Oppose moderately		00000000	00	
Oppose strongly			000	000

PERCENTAGE

Note: Each 0 = 1 percent.

Source: Constructed by the author.

FIGURE 4.7

Attitudes toward a Policy of Stressing Early Pregnancy Tests, Southern City, 1977

	Policy Makers (N = 62)	Service Providers (N = 55)	Adult General Public (N = 309)	Teenage Mothers (N = 35)
Favor strongly	0000000000 0000000000 0000000000 0000000000 0000000000 0000000000 0000000000 0000000000 00	0000000000 0000000000 0000000000 0000000000 0000000000 0000000000 0000000000 0000000000 00000	0000000000 0000000000 0000000000 0000000000 0000000000 0000000000 0000000000 0000000000 0000	0000000000 0000000000 0000000000 0000000000 0000000000 0000000000 0000000000 000000
Favor moderately	0000000000 000000	0000000000 00	0000000000 000	0000000000
Not sure	00	000	00	000
Oppose moderately				
Oppose strongly			0	0000000000 00

PERCENTAGE

Note: Each 0 = 1 percent.

Source: Constructed by the author.

FIGURE 4.8

State and Federal Decision Makers' Attitudes toward a Policy of Stressing Early Pregnancy Tests, 1977

PERCENTAGE

	North Carolina Judges (N = 125)	North Carolina Legislators (N = 101)	North Carolina HSAs (N = 58)	U.S. Congressmen (N = 83)	U.S. HEW* (N = 43)
Favor strongly	0000000000 0000000000 0000000000 0000000000 0000000000 0000000000 000000000	0000000000 0000000000 0000000000 0000000000 0000000000 0000000000 0000	0000000000 0000000000 0000000000 0000000000 0000000000 0000000000 0000000000 0000	0000000000 0000000000 0000000000 0000000000 0000000000 000000000	0000000000 0000000000 0000000000 0000000000 0000000000 0000000000 0000000000 0000000000 0000000000 000000
Favor moderately	0000000000 00000	0000000000 0000000000	0000	0000000000 0000000000 000	00
Not sure	0000	0000	00	0000000	00
Oppose moderately	00	00		0	

*Human services administrators in the U.S. Department of Health, Education and Welfare.

Note: Each 0 = 1 percent.

Source: Constructed by the author.

FIGURE 4.9

Attitudes toward a Local Policy of Talking with Pregnant Teenagers about All Alternatives, Farmville, 1977

	Policy Makers (N = 63)	Service Providers (N = 54)	Adult General Public (N = 313)	Teenage Mothers (N = 35)
Favor strongly	0000000000 0000000000 0000000000 0000000000 0000000000 0000000000 0000000000 00000	0000000000 0000000000 0000000000 0000000000 0000000000 0000000000 0000000000 0000000000 0	0000000000 0000000000 0000000000 0000000000 0000000000 0000000000 000000	0000000000 0000000000 0000000000 0000000000 0000000000 000000
Favor moderately	0000000000 0000000000	0000000000 000	0000000000 0000	0000000000 0000000000
Not sure	0000	000	0000000	0000000000 0000000000
Oppose moderately			00	000000
Oppose strongly	00	000	0	

Note: Each 0 = 1 percent.

Source: Constructed by the author.

81

FIGURE 4.10

Attitudes toward a Local Policy of Talking about All Alternatives with Pregnant Teenagers, Southern City, 1977

	Policy Makers (N = 62)	Service Providers (N = 55)	Adult General Public (N = 309)	Teenage Mothers (N = 35)
Favor strongly	0000000000 0000000000 0000000000 0000000000 0000000000 0000000000 0000000000 0000000000 0000	0000000000 0000000000 0000000000 0000000000 0000000000 0000000000 0000000000 0000000000 0000000000 0	0000000000 0000000000 0000000000 0000000000 0000000000 0000000000 0000000000 0000000000 00000	0000000000 0000000000 0000000000 0000000000 0000000000 0000000000 0000000
Favor moderately	00000000	000000000	000000000	0000000000 00000
Not sure	00000		0000	0000000000 00
Oppose moderately	000		0	
Oppose strongly			0	000000

PERCENTAGE

Note: Each 0 = 1 percent.

Source: Constructed by the author.

FIGURE 4.11

State and Federal Decision Makers' Attitudes toward a Policy of Talking about All Alternatives with Pregnant Teenagers, 1977

	North Carolina Judges (N = 125)	North Carolina Legislators (N = 101)	North Carolina HSAs (N = 58)	U.S. Congress-men (N = 83)	U.S. HEW* (N = 43)
Favor strongly	0000000000 0000000000 0000000000 0000000000 0000000000 0000000000 0000000000 0	0000000000 0000000000 0000000000 0000000000 0000000000 0000	0000000000 0000000000 0000000000 0000000000 0000000000 0000000000 0000000000 00	0000000000 0000000000 0000000000 0000000000 0000000000 000	0000000000 0000000000 0000000000 0000000000 0000000000 0000000000 0000000000 0000000000 000
Favor moderately	0000000000 00	0000000000 0000000000 000000000	000000	0000000000 000000000	0000000
Not sure	000000	00000	00	00000	
Oppose moderately		00		0	
Oppose strongly	0			00	

*Human services administrators in the U.S. Department of Health, Education and Welfare.

Note: Each 0 = 1 percent.

Source: Constructed by the author.

83

On the question of whether, as a regular policy, service agencies should discuss abortion, adoption, keeping the child with marriage, and keeping the child without marriage, there was nearly unanimous agreement across the respondent groups. As Figures 4.9-4.11 show, 90 percent of the respondents favored teenagers' being presented with all of these solutions as acceptable alternative ways to manage their pregnancy. This feeling that the policy ought to be presented in an unbiased manner seemed to appeal to nearly all persons in the community.

SUMMARY

Southern City policy makers and service providers have made pregnancy tests readily available to teenagers. Farmville policy makers and service providers have permitted pregnancy tests to be difficult to obtain except through private physicians' offices. Southern City offers a large array of counseling sources that appear to be used by teenagers. In contrast, little effective pregnancy counseling is available to Farmville teenagers.

Policy makers, service providers, the general public, and teenage mothers in both communities overwhelmingly supported policies of stressing a need for early pregnancy tests and for talking with pregnant teenagers about all options. Similarly overwhelming support for both pregnancy testing and discussing all options was demonstrated among all state- and federal-level respondents.

We began this chapter by observing that one of the measures of community attitudes toward human sexuality is the degree to which pregnancy tests are made available or unavailable, easy or hard to get. We have shown that Southern City makes pregnancy tests easy to get, while Farmville makes them hard to get. We turn now to another major indicator of community attitudes toward human sexuality: teen access to abortions.

5

TEEN ABORTIONS IN
FARMVILLE AND
SOUTHERN CITY

I do not believe any doctor in Farmville would perform
an abortion. I think most girls go to Beaufort. There
was a fine doctor at the Public Health Department about
four years ago who came intermittently from Beaufort
who gave advice on and, in fact, did do abortions, but
he worked in Beaufort.

> Observations of a
> 40-year-old Farmville mother

The situation is not nearly as bleak as the Farmville housewife
believes it to be, since there are numerous doctors in both Farmville
and Southern City who perform abortions. Our data show abortion to
be readily available in both communities to any teenagers who persist
in actively seeking it and are either able to pay for it themselves or
qualify for public abortion funds made available locally despite a federal ban.

THE GEOGRAPHY OF ABORTION SEEKING

Private physicians in both communities showed no unwillingness
to perform abortions or to make referrals to physicians who do. Even
so, as Figure 5.1 shows, two-thirds of the Farmville women who obtained abortions in 1976 chose to go outside the county. The majority
of women obtaining abortions outside Farmville went to the large,
publicly supported hospital nearby in Beaufort (25 percent of the time)
or to abortion clinics that advertise in the Farmville newspaper (11
percent of the time), or to Center County (22 percent of the time).

FIGURE 5.1

Percentages of Abortions by Location, Farmville and
Southern City, 1975 and 1976

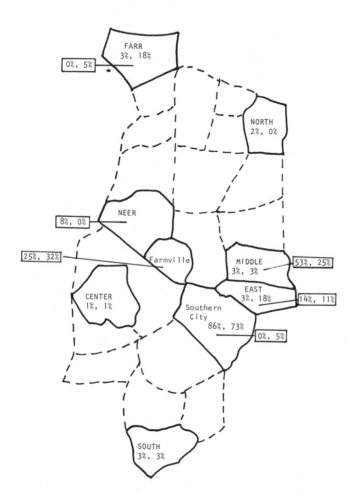

Note: Statistics for Southern City appear inside the county
lines; those for Farmville appear outside—1975 figures are given
first. Farmville abortions numbered 86 in 1975 and 106 in 1976.
Southern City abortions numbered 1,402 in 1975 and 1,764 in 1976.

Source: Data provided by North Carolina Department of Human
Resources, Division of Health Services, Public Health Statistics
Branch.

TABLE 5.1

Where Teenagers Seek Abortion Services: Views of Policy Makers,
Service Providers, and General Public, Farmville and Southern
City, 1977
(percent)

	Policy Makers		Service Providers		General Public	
	F	SC	F	SC	F	SC
Outside the community	57	9	69	26	48	13
Hospital	7	21	2	20	21	18
Private physician	28	16	21	9	14	10
Clinic	0	22	0	26	10	28
Public Health Department	3	19	1	11	3	16
Department of Mental Health	2	2	5	0	1	0
Department of Social Services	0	3	0	1	0	3
None available	0	0	0	0	2	4
Other	3	8	2	7	1	8
Total responses excluding don't know	60	64	86	90	178	164
Don't know	12	8	1	1	120	110
Total responses	72	72	87	91	298	274
Number	48	40	37	35	237	215

Note: F = Farmville; SC = Southern City.

Source: Compiled by the author.

Southern City residents, in contrast, chose to have 73 percent
of their abortions in their hometown hospitals and abortion clinics in
1976. In 1975, 86 percent of Southern City residents obtained their
abortions in their home community. As Figure 5.1 shows, 15 percent of those women using Southern City abortion facilities in 1975
shifted to a new clinic in East County in 1976. The East County clinic
has a reputation for sensitive care and offers early abortions for
$200.
    As Table 5.1 shows, the beliefs of Farmville residents about
the proportion of teenagers who seek abortions outside the community
ranged from the general public's estimate of 48 percent to the service
providers' estimate of 69 percent. Data are not available from each

of the institutions outside the community on the actual number of
Farmville teenagers who obtained abortions in the hospitals and abortion clinics in nearby counties, but the actual count data obtained from
General Hospital in nearby Beaufort suggest that the larger proportion
of Farmville women seeking abortion outside the community hospitals
are teenagers. Of the 27 residents of Farmville who obtained abortions at General Hospital in 1976, 19 (approximately 75 percent) were
teenagers (one aged 13, two aged 17, 3 each aged 14 and 19, five each
aged 15 and 18). Teenagers apparently seek the greater anonymity
offered by out-of-the-community abortion facilities. This impression
was shared by the few teens from the general public, who believed
67 percent of teenagers seek abortions "outside the county."

The responses recorded in Table 5.1 for Southern City accurately reflect the tendency for Southern City residents to seek abortions within their own community. Responses by policy makers, service providers, and the general public indicated an awareness of the
availability of abortion clinics, with estimates in a range of 14 to 28
percent for clinics as a source for abortions for teenagers. The service providers' estimate of the frequency with which Southern City
teenagers seek abortions outside the community was within two percentage points of the actual practice in the community. Views of policy makers and the general public reflected the situation of the previous year, when fewer residents of Southern City were being attracted
to the abortion clinic in nearby East County.

POLICY MAKERS' VIEWS ON THE
AVAILABILITY OF ABORTIONS

> So goddamn many [abortions] that hospital residents
> have no time.
>
> A physician on the
> mental health board in Farmville

Most Farmville county commissioners and city councilmen have
not thought much about the issue of teenage access to abortion. Aside
from three who said they did not know, responses were "You've got
me," or "Well, I would say Beaufort or James University," or "I've
heard of one in Center County," or "There's several places in Virginia, costs $200." One policy maker stated that the "only way is if
you go to the family doctor . . . I don't know of any M.D. doing it
without parental consent." Named influentials in Farmville were
somewhat better informed. Two said they did not know, four named
actual possible sources in and outside the county, and one responded
that there "used to be a guy in the textile industry for $50." Mental

health board members were generally well informed, mentioning General Hospital in Beaufort most often. A physician member commented, "General Hospital is doing so goddamn many that hospital residents have no time." This physician added, "Physicians don't refer girls to clinics (they're not treated very well, and the experience is likely to be traumatic)." None of the three mental health board members in Farmville knew of any place to obtain abortions. Some Farmville school board members viewed the teenagers as seeking anonymity by going outside the county ("Farmville's being a small place, it would be very hard to go to the local hospital and keep it quiet"), while other board members thought teenagers openly walk into the local hospital and ask for abortions.

The information level among the Southern City policy makers varied widely. One very surprising response: five of the seven health board members did not know where teenage women in their community go to seek abortions. Neither of the Department of Social Services board members knew of any source for abortion services for teenagers. Two of the generally well-informed members of the mental health board pointed to differences in abortion-related behavior depending on socioeconomic status. One replied, "I do not know where the poor girls go. The rich girls are sent away for abortions with the knowledge of their parents." A second mental health board member commented that whether abortion is sought inside or outside the county depends on socioeconomic status "and how much secrecy is sought." Seven of the ten school board members knew of specific local sources for abortions for teenagers; three knew of no sources.

FARMVILLE SERVICE PROVIDERS' VIEWS ON THE AVAILABILITY OF ABORTIONS

The predominant impression gained from studying Farmville service providers was one of random information levels and interests. There was no pattern of abortion information levels available to teenagers who become pregnant. What a pregnant girl was told about abortion costs and services and what counseling help she received were random events based on the person she happened to contact. Clearly there is no one source of information to which the teenagers in Farmville are referred. If they go to the Health Department, they are given some telephone numbers in several counties around the state. Beyond that, teens generally are on their own. Our general impression was that teenagers who become pregnant are not scolded, but neither do they get much information or sympathy. The response seems to be along the line of "You have a problem—that's too bad. Here are some telephone numbers. We hope you can work it out."

The service providers play the key role in determining the conditions under which teenagers in the two communities seek services related to abortion. The staff of the Farmville Health Department was well informed about possible sources to which to refer teenagers who came to them for help. Some, they said, were referred to private physicians in Farmville, "but the majority won't do it in Farmville because people know everyone." Beaufort was seen as the place to refer those teenagers who were underage. If the teenager had money and did not want her parents to know about her pregnancy, she was referred to the East County clinic or to nearby Carolina Women's Clinic. At Beaufort's General Hospital the bill was about $375. If the teenager went to Center County, the bill was usually about $175. The Health Department personnel provided telephone numbers, but in Farmville the teenager must take the initiative from there.

Farmville physicians were uniformly aware of the hospitals and clinics in surrounding counties that do abortions, and apparently would refer a teenager to a nearby county if she wished to avoid having an abortion in the Farmville Hospital. The members of the mental health center staff were generally aware that abortions were available, but did not have immediate experiences with actually making referrals. One staff member commented that a psychiatrist working at the mental health center sometimes did psychiatric evaluations for teenagers and then sent them to General Hospital in Beaufort, but "I don't know if OB/GYN men in town do abortions in the hospital—I've never heard of it." If a Farmville teenager were to ask the local pharmacists for information about sources of abortion, three of the six would tell her only of sources outside the community, one would tell her to go to the local hospital, one would name sources inside and outside the county, and one would not know of any sources.

If teenagers approached the ten key school administrators we interviewed, five could tell them of places inside and outside the community, two would know only of places outside the community, and three would not know of any place. One of the latter, a school principal, replied, when asked where teenagers in his community go for abortions, "I wouldn't have any way of knowing that." One of the four school counselors we interviewed could tell a teenager of sources both inside and outside the community; one did not know of any sources.

By far the best and most uniformly informed service providers, with the exception of the physicians, were the social services workers. All those interviewed seem acquainted with abortion referral sources both inside and outside the community. The general view was expressed by one social worker: "Girls don't want to go to the local hospital because of gossip, even though transportation elsewhere is difficult."

SOUTHERN CITY SERVICE PROVIDERS'
VIEWS ON THE AVAILABILITY OF ABORTIONS

To compare the attitudes and information levels in Farmville
with the attitudes and information levels in Southern City is a study
in striking contrasts. The existence and acceptance of abortion in
Southern City was such that, in contrast with the random Farmville
respondents, the majority of Southern City respondents, among both
medical doctors and other service providers, distinguished between
abortion sources that offer first trimester abortion and those, such
as the medical center at James University, where only second trimester abortions are performed.

A second striking difference between Farmville and Southern
City was that service providers in Southern City were uniformly aware
of at least the two major sources of assistance: the Health Department and the Hayworth Clinic. Hayworth Clinic is operated by a concerned Southern City obstetrician who is sensitive to the counseling
and psychological needs of women patients, especially teenagers.
Knowledge of the Hayworth Clinic and the Health Department as centers to which to refer pregnant teenagers was present among nearly
all the service providers we studied. (The Health Department clinic
was mentioned by all the social services workers interviewed, by all
mental health personnel interviewed, by all pharmacists, by eight of
the ten school administrators, and by all school counselors.) This
fact might have been expected, given the uniformly well-informed responses by the Southern City service providers on the availability
and location of counseling and pregnancy testing services in Southern
City. However, the uniformity of this knowledge base among a wide
range of service providers is striking. All of the six key members
of the Health Department family planning staff mentioned six places
for abortion referral inside and outside the community. Their information was consistent from individual to individual.

The third striking difference between Farmville and Southern
City was in the approach and tone taken toward the pregnant teenager.
In Farmville the Health Department offered some telephone numbers
of clinics around the state and ended its involvement at that point.
Any teenager who went to the Health Department in Southern City for
help received three pamphlets that offer full information on sources
for abortion and convey nonjudgmental attitudes. The approach of the
Health Department is summed up at the beginning of one pamphlet:

> If you are pregnant and feel you are not ready for a baby
> now, there are several possibilities you can consider.
> We have enclosed information on maternity homes,
> adoption, and abortion for you to think about. It is very

helpful for a woman who is considering what to do about
an unwanted pregnancy to discuss her feelings with someone and to receive correct information on the kinds of help
available. When you receive the results of your pregnancy test, you will be referred to a counselor who will
help you with these needs. Some of the possible places
your counselor may refer you to for help are listed on
the following sheets.

If you are not pregnant and do not want a baby at this
time, it is important that you obtain a good method of
birth control and use it correctly. We have attached a
pamphlet on family planning methods and information on
where you can receive family planning aid for your use.

This brief pamphlet is reproduced in Appendix E. In it four
maternity homes in which charges are based on ability to pay are discussed. Five organizations offering help in putting a baby up for
adoption are listed, as are seven sources of family planning services.
Finally, seven abortion sources are discussed, with names and ad-
dresses, the types of procedures performed, the approximate cost
for each procedure at each center, and other information, such as
payment procedures, whether Medicaid stickers are accepted or not,
days and hours open. Each teenager in Southern City who contacted
the Health Department was also given a pamphlet from the Virginia
Medical Center for Women, a nonprofit corporation a few hours'
drive from Southern City. The pamphlet describes the center and
sets the tone in its opening paragraph:

> The Virginia Medical Center for Women was organized
> in 1973 by a gynecologist and a Presbyterian minister,
> who through working with several thousand patients since
> 1970, believe that the happiness and satisfaction that can
> come through a wanted and timely pregnancy has its
> counterpart in the women who face the unhappiness and
> sometimes tragedy of an unwanted pregnancy. The
> Clinic is committed to quality medical care, at as low a
> cost as possible.

Over half the teenagers who responded in the general public samples
in both communities, however, did not know where abortions could
be obtained by teenagers in their community. One ninth-grade male
in Southern City said, "None available." Of the 13 teenage respondents in Southern City, two mentioned Hayworth Clinic and only one
mentioned the Health Department. Among the eight teenage respondents in Farmville, five said they did not know, two mentioned the local

hospital, and one said "outside the county." As mentioned earlier, it was not possible to determine to what degree these few teenagers are similar to the entire teenage population in these two communities.

ABORTION TRENDS IN THE TWO COMMUNITIES

Increasing Proportions among Farmville Teenagers

From 1973 through 1976 the percentage of abortions performed on Farmville teenagers increased dramatically, while that for Southern City teenagers remained steady and small by comparison. The data in Tables 5.2 and 5.3 may be viewed in several ways. In Farmville the percentage of total abortions obtained by the teenagers rose each year, going from 45.5 percent of all abortions in 1973 to 48 percent in 1974, then to 49.6 percent of all abortions in 1976.

In Southern City the percentage of all abortions obtained by teenagers rose from 24.2 percent in 1973, to 36.1 percent in 1974, to 37.9 percent in 1975, then declined to 31.5 percent in 1976. The 1976 percentage of all abortions to residents accounted for by the teenage population is very different in the two communities: in Farmville teenagers accounted for 53 percent of all abortions to residents, while in Southern City they accounted for 31 percent (down from a high of 38 percent the year before). Abortion behaviors established a regular pattern during these years as legal abortions became both increasingly available and customary. The number of abortions to persons aged 20 and over in Farmville remained fairly constant over these years: 55 in 1973, 48 in 1974, and 53 in 1976. Abortions obtained by Southern City adults rose and fell, doubling during 1973-76 (603 in 1973, 909 in 1974, 870 in 1975, and 1,209 in 1976). The actual numbers and the age groups of persons obtaining abortions in the two communities seem subject to what might be normal fluctuations.

What is useful for our purposes is to look for long-term trends and differences in abortion statistics that maintain themselves over time and at different levels for these two communities. One such trend is the consistently high percentage of all abortions obtained by teenagers in Farmville, which becomes clear when one looks at the abortions obtained by adult women in the two communities. Older Farmville women obtained a smaller and smaller percentage of abortions in each of the years 1973 through 1976. Conversely, in Southern City the percentage of women aged 20 and over who obtained abortions always ranged in the sixtieth percentile (in Farmville it was the fiftieth percentile). In Farmville the percentage of abortions obtained by persons aged 20 and over ranged from 50.4 to 54.5 percent; in Southern City the percentage ranged from 62.1 to 68.5 percent. The result is that over the period 1973-76 an average of 12 to 15 percent more of the abortions among Farmville women were performed on teenagers.

TABLE 5.2

Number of Abortions Reported to the State, by Age and Race, Farmville,
1973/74 and 1976

| Year and Age | Race | | | Total | |
	White	Black	Not Stated	Number	Percent
1973					
14	0	2	0	2	2.3
15	0	4	0	4	4.5
16	4	3	0	7	6.8
17	2	2	0	4	4.5
18	14	4	0	18	18.2
19	4	5	0	9	9.1
Total teens	24	20	—	—	45.5
20 and over	30	23	2	55	54.5
Total	54	43	2	99	—
Percent	54.5	43.2	2.3	—	100.0
1974					
14	0	0	0	0	—
15	4	0	0	4	4.4
16	4	0	0	4	4.4
17	6	4	0	10	11.4
18	0	8	0	8	8.7
19	15	3	0	18	19.2
Total teens	29	15	—	—	48.0
20 and over	39	9	0	48	52.0
Total	68	24	0	92	—
Percent	73.9	26.1	0.0	—	100.0
1976					
14	0	0	0	0	—
15	6	8	0	14	13.3
16	13	4	0	17	15.7
17	6	0	2	8	7.7
18	4	5	0	9	8.1
19	5	0	0	5	4.8
Total teens	34	17	2	—	49.6
20 and over	84	19	0	53	50.4
Total	68	36	2	106	—
Percent	63.9	34.2	1.9	—	100.0

Source: Compiled by the author.

TABLE 5.3

Number of Abortions Reported to the State, by Age and Race, Southern City, 1973-76

Year and Age	Race			Total Number	Percent
	White	Black	Not Stated		
1973					
13	0	7	0	7	0.7
14	11	11	0	22	2.5
15	9	11	0	20	2.2
16	9	27	0	36	3.9
17	20	25	0	45	4.9
18	49	43	2	94	10.3
19	47	40	0	87	9.6
Total teens	145	164	2	311	24.2
20 and over	287	316	0	603	65.8
Total	432	480	2	914	—
Percent	47.2	52.6	0.2	—	100.0
1974					
13	0	6	0	6	0.4
14	9	3	0	12	0.9
15	24	25	0	49	3.5
16	47	21	0	68	4.7
17	50	27	0	77	5.4
18	121	34	0	155	10.9
19	89	57	0	146	10.3
Total teens	340	173	0	513	36.1
20 and over	598	308	3	909	64.0
Total	938	481	3	1,422	—
Percent	66.0	33.8	0.2	—	100.0
1975					
14	0	6	0	6	0.4
15	22	22	0	44	3.2
16	31	44	0	75	5.4
17	24	27	4	55	3.9
18	119	66	8	193	13.7
19	116	43	0	159	11.4
Total teens	312	208	12	532	37.9
20 and over	532	281	57	870	62.1
Total	844	489	69	1,402	—
Percent	60.2	34.8	5.0	—	100.0
1976					
13	0	4	0	4	0.2
14	0	9	0	9	0.5
15	46	20	1	67	3.8
16	42	28	3	73	4.1
17	55	25	0	80	4.5
18	102	34	1	137	7.8
19	104	72	2	178	10.1
Total teens	349	192	7	548	31.5
20 and over	772	376	69	1,209	68.5
Total	1,121	568	76	1,765	—
Percent	63.5	32.2	4.3	—	100.0

Source: Compiled by the author.

Increasing Proportions among White Teenagers

Another very clear trend from 1973 to 1976 was for the number of abortions to white teenagers to increase steadily in both communities while the number to black teenagers remained relatively stable. (See Table 5.4.) In Farmville the number of abortions to white teenagers rose from 24 in 1973 to 29 in 1974 and jumped to 42 in 1976, an increase of 75 percent over the period. During these same years the number of black teenagers in the two communities who obtained abortions remained at a relatively low and stable level. The number of reported abortions to black teenagers in Farmville varied from 20 in 1973 to 15 in 1974 to 17 in 1976. The number of black teenagers obtaining abortions in Southern City increased gradually, then decreased, ranging from 164 in 1973 to 192 in 1976.

TABLE 5.4

Number of Abortions to Women under Age 20, by Race, Farmville, Southern City, Multicounty Area, and North Carolina, 1973-76

	Farmville	Southern City	Multicounty Area	North Carolina
1973				
White	24	145	365	2,598
Black	20	164	442	1,489
1974				
White	29	340	604	4,222
Black	15	173	445	1,940
1975				
White	n.a.	312	697	5,117
Black	n.a.	208	575	2,284
1976				
White	42	349	764	5,639
Black	17	192	596	2,837

n.a. = not available

Source: Compiled from Tables 5.5, 5.8, and 5.9.

Increasing Proportions among
Younger Farmville Teenagers

Another long-term trend that was radically different for the two communities was the percentage of abortions for persons aged 15 to 17 in the two communities. A constantly higher percentage of abortions was performed on Farmville girls aged 15 to 17, trending upward from 16 percent of all abortions in that community in 1973 to an as yet unexplained 38 percent in 1976. In contrast, the percentage of abortions to persons aged 15 to 17 in Southern City remained relatively

FIGURE 5.2

Percentage of All Abortions Obtained by Women Aged 15 to 17,
Farmville, Southern City, and North Carolina, 1973-76

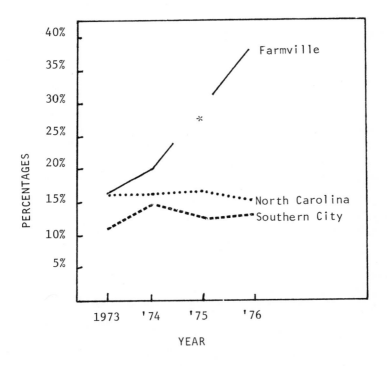

*1975 Farmville data not available.

Source: Derived from Table 5.6.

TABLE 5.5

Number of Abortions Reported to the State, by Age and Race, Multicounty Health Systems Agency Region, 1973-76

| Year and Age | Race | | | Total | |
	White	Black	Not Stated	Number	Percent
1973					
11	0	2	0	2	0.1
12	0	0	0	0	0.0
13	2	11	0	13	0.5
14	20	29	0	49	2.0
15	18	45	0	63	2.5
16	38	74	2	114	4.6
17	63	74	0	137	5.5
18	116	96	2	214	8.5
19	108	111	0	219	8.7
20 and over	861	831	7	1,699	67.7
Total	1,226	1,273	11	2,510	—
Percent	48.8	50.7	0.4	—	100.0
1974					
11	0	0	0	0	0.0
12	0	1	0	1	0.0
13	6	25	0	31	1.0
14	28	24	0	52	1.7
15	38	46	0	84	2.7
16	82	35	0	117	3.7
17	107	76	0	183	5.8
18	183	105	0	288	9.2
19	160	133	0	293	9.3
20 and over	1,221	856	6	2,083	66.6
Total	1,825	1,301	6	3,132	—
Percent	58.2	41.6	0.2	—	100.0
1975					
11	0	4	0	4	0.1
12	0	0	0	0	0.0
13	1	5	0	6	0.2
14	9	34	0	43	1.2
15	67	39	0	106	3.0
16	78	93	0	171	4.9
17	65	107	4	176	5.0
18	236	147	9	392	11.1
19	241	146	0	387	11.0
20 and over	1,322	837	69	2,228	63.5
Total	2,019	1,412	82	3,513	—
Percent	57.5	40.2	2.3	—	100.0
1976					
11	0	0	0	0	0.0
12	1	8	0	9	0.2
13	4	5	0	9	0.2
14	13	32	0	45	1.0
15	61	70	1	132	3.0
16	106	99	3	208	4.8
17	115	76	6	197	4.5
18	230	132	2	364	8.4
19	234	174	3	411	9.4
20 and over	1,666	1,238	76	2,980	68.4
Total	2,430	1,834	91	4,355	—
Percent	55.8	42.1	2.1	—	100.0

Source: North Carolina Department of Human Resources, Division of Health Services, Public Health Statistics Department.

TABLE 5.6

Number of Abortions Reported to the State, by Age and Race, North Carolina, 1973-76

	Race			Total	
Year and Age	White	Black	Not Stated	Number	Percent
1973					
10	0	2	0	2	0.0
11	4	7	0	11	0.1
12	0	7	0	7	0.1
13	13	54	0	67	0.6
14	90	94	0	184	1.5
15	267	150	2	419	3.5
16	424	247	4	675	5.7
17	534	253	0	787	6.6
18	671	330	7	1,008	8.4
19	595	345	0	940	7.9
20 and over	5,073	2,744	18	7,835	65.6
Total	7,671	4,233	31	11,935	—
Percent	64.3	35.5	0.3	—	100.0
1974					
11	0	3	0	3	0.0
12	4	8	0	12	0.1
13	31	58	0	89	0.5
14	163	121	0	284	1.7
15	364	190	0	554	3.4
16	665	260	5	930	5.6
17	794	339	7	1,140	6.9
18	1,204	473	2	1,681	10.2
19	997	488	1	1,486	9.0
20 and over	6,727	3,424	133	10,284	62.6
Total	10,949	5,364	150	16,463	—
Percent	66.5	32.6	0.9	—	100.0
1975					
11	4	4	0	8	0.0
12	4	17	0	21	0.1
13	41	45	0	86	0.4
14	134	122	5	261	1.3
15	413	247	0	660	3.3
16	813	345	13	1,171	5.9
17	895	373	19	1,287	6.4
18	1,582	580	31	2,193	11.0
19	1,231	551	0	1,782	8.9
20 and over	8,048	4,266	177	12,437	62.7
Total	13,165	6,550	245	19,960	—
Percent	66.0	32.8	1.2	—	100.0
1976					
11	1	1	0	2	0.0
12	2	19	0	21	0.1
13	19	62	0	81	0.3
14	149	165	8	322	1.4
15	415	303	5	723	3.1
16	802	421	11	1,234	5.2
17	1,005	474	15	1,494	6.3
18	1,753	630	14	2,397	10.3
19	1,493	762	6	2,261	9.6
20 and over	9,319	5,489	218	15,026	63.7
Total	14,958	8,326	277	23,561	—
Percent	63.5	35.3	1.2	—	100.0

Source: North Carolina Department of Human Resources, Division of Health Services, Public Health Statistics Department.

FIGURE 5.3

Abortion Rates, by Race for Women Aged 15 to 19, Farmville and
Southern City, 1973-76

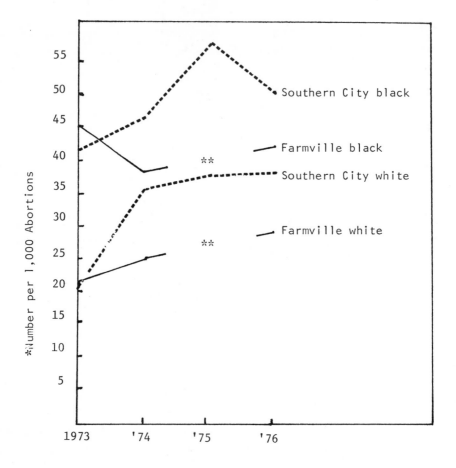

*1975 Farmville data not available.

Note: Abortion rate is number of abortions per 1,000 women.

Source: Constructed by the author.

FIGURE 5.4

Abortion Rates, by Race, for Women Aged 15 to 19, Farmville,
Southern City, and North Carolina, 1976

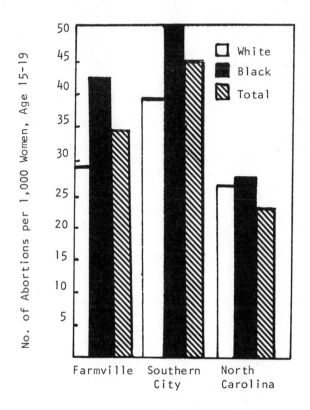

Note: Abortion rate is number of abortions per 1,000 women.

Source: Constructed by the author.

stable and at a significantly lower level of all abortions, ranging from
11 percent in 1973 to 13 percent in 1976 (see Figure 5.2).

Tables 5.5 and 5.6 provide comparative profiles of abortions
obtained in 1973-76 by residents in the multicounty health systems
agency area (Table 5.5) and in the state of North Carolina (Table 5.6).
Data from the multicounty area and the state resemble Southern City
data much more than Farmville data. (A summary of the characteristics of all women receiving abortions in North Carolina in 1976 appears in Appendix F.)

Because the black population is less than a quarter of the white
population, it becomes desirable to convert the number of births to

blacks and to whites in the two communities into abortion rates and abortion ratios. The abortion rate is the reported number of induced abortions per 1,000 women. A steady increase in the rate at which white women aged 15 to 19 obtained abortions from 1973 to 1976 can be seen in Figure 5.3, which shows a clear increase for Southern City white teenagers. In 1973 the rate at which black teenagers were obtaining abortions was more than double that of white teenagers. At the end of this four-year period in Farmville, the rate at which black teenagers obtained abortions had decreased by 7 percent. The total abortion rate for Farmville continued to rise over the four years because of the preponderance of whites in the population, which weighted the average toward the white abortion rate. If one takes the North Carolina abortion rates and the United States abortion rates into account, it becomes apparent that the rates at which Farmville teenagers, both black and white, were obtaining abortions were higher than the state or national average. During 1973-76 the abortion rates for Southern City teenagers rose by 90 percent, in contrast with the 38 percent rise in Farmville, ending up 9 percent higher than the Farmville rate. The rate at which black teenagers in Southern City obtained abortions began two-thirds higher than the rate of their counterparts in Farmville, and rose 22 percent over the four-year period, having peaked in 1975. The abortion rate for black teenagers in Southern City remained 47 percent higher than that for black teenagers in Farmville in 1976. Figure 5.4 gives comparative data for 1976.

SERVICE GAPS

> Society has changed—it doesn't happen just to trash anymore, but finer people, too—they use their family physician and other options.
>   A Farmville county commissioner

A way to measure the level or prevalence of abortions, besides calculating the abortion rates, is the abortion ratio, which is the reported number of abortions per 1,000 live births. This is a much more useful indicator on prevalence of abortion. The abortion ratio can be thought of as a measure of efficiency with which teenagers are managing their sexuality. In Chapter 6, in which we describe and discuss the contraceptive successes and failures of teenagers in the two communities, we report that no more than 26 percent of the teenagers who gave birth in 1976 in Farmville and Southern City had any intention or desire to become pregnant when they did. Given this, the information provided by calculating the abortion ratios for the communities gives some startling indications of the inability of teenagers to manage fertility without having unintended pregnancies.

FIGURE 5.5

Abortion Ratio, by Race, for Women Aged 15 to 19, Farmville,
Southern City, and North Carolina, 1976

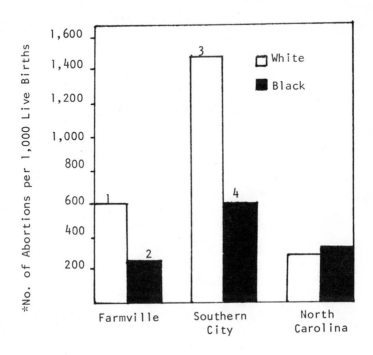

1 = 34 abortions; 56 live births reported
2 = 17 abortions; 65 live births reported
3 = 349 abortions; 234 live births reported
4 = 179 abortions; 302 live births reported

Note: Abortion ratio is number of abortions per 1,000 live births.

Source: Constructed by the author.

For every 1,000 live births to teenagers aged 15 to 19 in Farmville, white teenagers between those ages obtained 607 abortions at
the 1976 rate (see Figure 5.5). Black teenagers obtained considerably fewer—261 abortions per 1,000 live births. Southern City white
teenagers obtained abortions at a rate of 1,491 in 1976; blacks, at a
rate of 592. A sharp contrast existed between the two communities
among both racial groups. White teenagers in Southern City obtained
abortions at a rate 146 percent higher than the rate of white teenagers
in Farmville in 1976. Black teenagers in Southern City obtained abor-

TABLE 5.7

Legal Abortion Ratios by Age, Selected States, 1974

State*	15	15 to 19	20 to 24	25 to 29	30 to 34	35 to 39	40	Total
California	2,641	884	396	271	330	516	685	447
Connecticut	1,395	599	244	153	176	306	514	255
District of Columbia	1,437	1,190	1,159	991	903	1,200	1,754	1,115
Georgia	635	347	245	194	233	359	414	265
Illinois	379	287	195	127	176	300	520	197
Kentucky	1,031	159	80	59	53	67	74	93
Mississippi	7	3	3	2	4	6	9	3
New Hampshire	846	151	47	27	41	79	157	58
New York	2,749	1,308	659	416	553	917	1,566	675
City	3,458	1,859	1,116	797	970	1,394	2,274	1,138
Upstate	1,827	788	291	143	221	458	928	306
North Carolina	772	279	161	126	192	310	552	195
Pennsylvania	1,549	509	245	131	189	306	490	258
South Carolina	245	102	73	54	82	107	165	80
Tennessee	389	175	94	69	95	108	153	110
Virginia	1,068	384	192	113	146	266	492	210
Total	1,156	491	263	184	244	389	585	292

*Live births are based on 1973 distributions of live births, by age of mother, from each state health agency.

Note: Abortion ratios are calculated as the number of legal abortions for women of a given age group per 1,000 live births to women of the same age group. ("Unknown" age for each state is redistributed according to known age distribution of that state.) Live births by age of mother are from state health agencies unless otherwise noted.

Source: U.S., Department of Health, Education and Welfare, Abortion Surveillance, 1974 (Atlanta: Center for Disease Control, 1976), table 6, p. 20.

tions at a rate 126 percent above that of Farmville black teenagers. One result of the tremëndous unevenness in rates between Farmville and Southern City was that black teenagers in Southern City obtained abortions in 1976 at a rate nearly equal to the rate of abortions obtained by white teenagers in Farmville.

When abortion ratios for selected states in 1974 (the latest available data) are compared with those of Southern City, the latter are seen to be higher than those of any selected state and higher than that of Washington, D.C. (see Table 5.7). State abortion ratios are diluted by the inclusion of rural areas and city areas in which there are few services. Thus, New York City and Washington, D.C., are the only fully comparable areas for our purposes, because it can be assumed that a number of large cities had high abortion rates that are masked by the inclusion of data from throughout the state. In addition, the abortion ratio most likely went up during 1975 and 1976. Nevertheless, the Southern City abortion ratios appear to be among the very highest in the nation, assuming that New York City and Washington, D.C., are among the best served areas in the United States. The abortion ratios for Farmville are exceeded only by that of California (884 in 1974, compared with 868 in Farmville in 1976).

Legal abortion ratios are highest in the 14-and-younger age group. We have not attempted to calculate these data for Farmville and Southern City because the numbers are too small to be meaningful when projected to the rates per 1,000. The abortion ratios clearly are highest for the 19-and-under age group, decrease through the twenties, then increase again in the late thirties and forties.

In order to illustrate the magnitude of the social costs of the way Farmville and Southern City currently manage adolescent fertility, we have calculated the number and immediate medical costs of abortions and unwanted births per 1,000 babies wanted by young women aged 15 to 19 in Farmville and Southern City. In Farmville in 1976, 24 percent of the teenagers who gave birth wanted to get pregnant; in Southern City, 26 percent. Some of these teenagers were married and clearly sought to have a child at that point in life. We have not attempted to break down the data into births to married and unmarried women because numbers are too small to be satisfactory for these purposes. The costs of achieving 1,000 wanted births to teenagers in these two communities can be grasped by studying Table 5.8. Here we have calculated the number of unwanted live births and the number of abortions necessary to result in 1,000 wanted births to teenagers in Farmville as 3,166 unwanted births and 3,658 abortions. Thus, 3,166 unwanted births and 3,658 abortions, a total of at least 6,824 more pregnancies than were intended, occur along with every 1,000 births wanted by teenagers in Farmville. In Southern City 2,846 unwanted births and 7,934 abortions occur along with every 1,000 wanted

TABLE 5.8

Number and Immediate Medical Costs of Abortions and Unwanted Births per 1,000 Babies Wanted by Young Women Aged 15 to 19, Farmville and Southern City, 1976

Events for Each 1,000 Actual Births	Multiplier for 1,000 Wanted Births		Unwanted Births and Abortions	Immediate Medical Costs (prenatal and delivery) per 1,000 Wanted Births (dollars)		
Farmville						
Wanted 240						
Unwanted (probably) 60	× 4.166	=	250	× 1,250	=	312,500
Unwanted (definitely) 700	× 4.166	=	2,916	× 1,250	=	3,645,000
Total unwanted births			3,166			
Reported abortions 878	× 4.166	=	3,658	× 200	=	731,600
Total unwanted births and abortions			6,824			4,689,100
Southern City						
Wanted 260						
Unwanted (probably) 90	× 3.846	=	346	× 1,250	=	432,500
Unwanted (definitely) 650	× 3.846	=	2,500	× 1,250	=	3,125,000
Total unwanted births			2,846			
Reported abortions 2,063	× 3.846	=	7,934	× 200	=	1,586,800
Total unwanted births and abortions			10,780			5,144,300

Note: To convert the 24 percent rate of births wanted in Southern City and the 26 percent rate of births wanted in Farmville to a common rate per 1,000 wanted births, the multipliers are 240 X 4.166 = 1,000 and 260 X 3,846 = 1,000.

Source: Compiled by the author.

births. In all, at the 1976 rates, 10,780 unwanted pregnancies in addition to the 1,000 wanted pregnancies must occur each time 1,000 wanted babies are born to Southern City teenagers.

We argue that the 2,846 unwanted births and the 7,934 abortions in Southern City represent unmet fertility management needs. We will explore the rationale and value assumptions behind this estimate of unmet need at the beginning of Chapter 6.

Medical costs associated with either abortion or prenatal care and delivery, which are in addition to costs of the 1,000 wanted births, amount to approximately $4,689,100 in Farmville and $5,144,300 in Southern City for each 1,000 wanted births to teenagers. The social and personal costs of these abortions and births will be examined below, in the discussion of value gaps that exist between the policies set by the American Public Health Association (APHA) and respondents in these two communities.

VALUE GAPS

The value judgments made in the APHA policies are without qualification. The APHA mades the value judgment that "Adolescents must be provided access to . . . abortion . . . without parental consent." In the minds of a number of people this may be regarded as an extreme position. To test the degree of value congruence with the recommended APHA standard of abortion for any teenager without parental consent, we asked several questions in our research instruments. We constructed a scale from the five questions (out of 20 in one instrument) that were focused on abortion. One that involved providing program funding for abortion and contraceptives will be discussed in Chapter 6, which focuses on contraception for teenagers. In this chapter we discuss the two questions we asked first, about simply making abortion available to teenagers and making abortion available without parental consent. Thus, through direct questions and scaling we have developed a profile of respondents' values surrounding the provision of abortion to teenagers. Two broad trends are evident: Farmville is consistently more conservative than Southern City and service providers are consistently the most supportive group affirming a need for abortion services for teenagers. A number of other identifiable trends are discussed below.

FIGURE 5.6

Attitudes of Policy Makers, Service Providers, Adult General Public, and Teenage Mothers toward a Policy of Making Abortion Available to Teenagers, Farmville, 1977

	Policy Makers (N = 63)	Service Providers (N = 54)	Adult General Public (N = 313)	Teenage Mothers (N = 35)
Favor strongly	0000000000 0000000	0000000000 0000000000 0000000000 0000000000 000000	0000000000 000000	0000000000 00000000
Favor moderately	0000000000 0000000000 0000000000 0000	0000000000 0000000000 0000000000 00000	0000000000 00000000	0000000000 00000
Not sure	0000000000 000000000	0000000000 0	0000000000 000000	0000000000 0000000000 00000
Oppose moderately	0000000000 0000000	000	0000000000 000	0000000000 00000000
Oppose strongly	0000000000 000	00000	0000000000 0000000000 0000000000 0000000	0000000000 0000000000 0000

Note: Each 0 = 1 percent.

Source: Constructed by the author.

FIGURE 5.7

Attitudes of Policy Makers, Service Providers, Adult General Public, and Teenage Mothers toward a Policy of Making Abortion Available to Teenagers, Southern City, 1977

PERCENTAGE

	Policy Makers (N = 62)	Service Providers (N = 55)	Adult General Public (N = 309)	Teenage Mothers (N = 35)
Favor strongly	0000000000 0000000000 0000000000 0000000000 0000000000 000	0000000000 0000000000 0000000000 0000000000 0000000000 0000000000 00000000	0000000000 0000000000 0000000000 00000	0000000000 0000000000 0
Favor moderately	0000000000 0000000000 0	0000000000 0000000000 0000	0000000000 0000000000 000000	0000000000 00000000
Not sure	0000000000 000000	0000000000 00000	0000000000 00000	0000000000 0000000000 000⁻
Oppose moderately	00000000	000	000000	0000000000
Oppose strongly	00		0000000000 00000000	0000000000 0000000000 000000000

Note: Each 0 = 1 percent.

Source: Compiled by the author.

109

POLICY MAKERS' VIEWS

In Southern City only 10 percent of policy makers either moderately or strongly opposed making abortions available to teenagers. In Farmville the proportion of policy makers opposing making abortion available to teenagers rose to 30 percent. Does this mean surprisingly high acceptance of abortion, or does it mean low acceptance? These figures are difficult to interpret satisfactorily for all readers. Depending on the assumptions that one holds concerning the availability of abortion in the United States, one can reach various conclusions from the data given in Figures 5.6 and 5.7. Our interpretation is necessarily based on our own judgments about what these figures mean in the context of the current debate over abortion in the United States. The reader may come to other conclusions from studying the data.

We believe there is an atmosphere of conservatism about abortion for teenagers in Farmville when Farmville attitudes are compared with Southern City attitudes. However, when Farmville attitudes are examined on their own, there seems to be little serious opposition to abortion for teenagers among the policy makers. The slightly more than 10 percent of policy makers strongly opposed to providing abortions for teenagers reflects weak opposition. Support for abortion for teenagers is even stronger in Southern City. Depending on one's reading of the politics of community policy making, there appears to be at least moderate support among policy makers in Farmville and strong support among Southern City policy makers for making abortion available to teenagers. About half the policy makers in Farmville and three-fourths of the policy makers in Southern City support the policy idea.

SERVICE PROVIDERS' VIEWS

Service providers in both communities strongly support a policy of making abortion available to teenagers. Few service providers in either community (8 percent in Farmville and 3 percent in Southern City) are either moderately or strongly opposed to such a policy. Much stronger support for the APHA's proposed policies by service providers than by the other groups is evident in views on most of the issues covered by the policies for care. This is not surprising, since the proposed policies were mostly written by service providers. A clear trend throughout our data was for service providers to be consistently more in favor of the APHA policies than the general public or the policy makers were.

We believe there is a direct correlation between the degree of closeness to the problem of pregnancies among teenagers and the types of policies one favors to solve the problem. Service providers come into direct contact with pregnant teenagers and their problems, whereas policy makers seldom actually confront the situation. The general public has even less direct contact with problem pregnancies than do the policy makers. In short, the willingness of respondents to have abortion made available to teenagers is directly correlated with the degree of contact they have with the problem and its impacts on teenagers.

DEGREE OF FAVORABILITY

Policy Makers

In order to get another perspective on the data, we constructed a scale consisting of five questions. Each question favors offering progressively more access to abortion for teenagers. (See Figure 5.8 for results and the bottom of the figure for the questions used.) Figure 5.8 measures the degree of favorableness toward a community policy of making abortion available to teenagers. Policy makers in Southern City were about twice as willing to have teenagers given access to abortion as Farmville policy makers were. Service providers in both communities, on the other hand, tended to be more favorable toward availability of abortion for teenagers. To the degree that this scale is predictive, one would expect that policies favoring abortion would be twice as likely to be developed in Southern City as in Farmville. Farmville policy makers would be unlikely to make a set of policies affirming teenagers' rights to access to abortion, whereas in Southern City one might predict that the key boards (public health, social services, mental health, school) would be likely to adopt policies similar to those of the APHA.

Service Providers

The situation regarding the service providers in the two communities is similar. In Farmville several of the key service provider boards or groups seemed unlikely to favor a policy of full access to abortions for teenagers. For example, in Farmville the private physicians were extremely influential in policy-making matters in the area of health, and only 29 percent of them (compared with 64 percent of the physicians in Southern City) favored a total of either four or five of the policy ideas. Ministers, too, were influential service providers and policy makers in Farmville, and only 36 percent of them scored high on the scale. School administrators scored similarly low in Farmville compared with school administrators in Southern City.

FIGURE 5.8

Percentages of Policy Makers and Service Providers Who Were Liberal on Four and Five Items of the Composite Abortion Attitude Scale, Farmville and Southern City, 1976

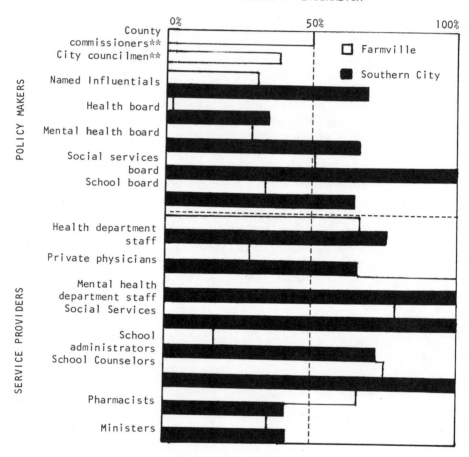

Scale:
Question 3, refusing abortion to anyone under 18
Question 6, talking about all alternatives, including abortion, with teenagers
Question 7, encouraging teenager to have the child
Question 13, making abortion available to teenagers
Question 17, allowing abortion without parental consent

*Not applicable for Southern City.

Source: Constructed by the author.

One might expect support for strong policies of providing access to abortion for teenagers from all service provider groups in Southern City except the pharmacists and ministers. In contrast, in Farmville key community support for this policy seemed unlikely to come from the ministers, physicians, and school administrators. The lack of support from these key persons in Farmville would make it difficult for the service provider groups favoring such a policy to act. Mental health, social services, and Health Department staffs supported the idea of abortion for teenagers, but apparently lacked strong support from key policy makers on their own and other boards; similarly, they lacked needed support from ministers, physicians, and school administrators. The extent to which actual policies on the provision of abortion services to teenagers are made by service providers, and the extent to which such policies are made by board members, probably will vary in every case and over time.

Certainly it is interesting to see that in Southern City the Health Department staff and the Health Department board both scored low on the scale. Normally this would be a reason to hold the scale suspect. In this specific situation the scale may be accurate, despite the apparent contradictory data on the Southern City Health Department board and service staff, because of the leadership and dedication of the Health Department director, who for several years has managed the family planning program.

General Public

Policy makers and service providers in the two communities seemed to reflect accurately the attitudes of the general public in these two communities. The general public in Southern City was twice as favorable as the general public in Farmville toward a policy of providing abortions for teenagers in their community. There was, then, a consistent theme of acceptability for this policy among the policy makers, service providers, and the general public in Southern City. Conversely, there was measurably less acceptance of a policy favoring abortion for teenagers in Farmville. About twice as many Farmville persons as Southern City persons strongly opposed the idea.

Cross Tabulations of Demographic Factors

We conducted an extensive series of cross tabulations to discover the sources of opposition to the provision of abortions for teenagers; we cross-tabulated age, sex, marital status, number of chil-

FIGURE 5.9

Attitudes of General Public, by Occupation, toward a City Policy of Making Abortion Available to Teenagers, Southern City, 1977

	Profes- sional (N = 45)	Mana- gerial (N = 42)	Clerical (N = 28)	Service (N = 23)	Blue Collar (N = 9)	Unem- ployed (N = 68)
Favor strongly	0000000000 0000000000 0000000000 0000000000 0000000000 000000	0000000000 0000000000 0000000000 0	0000000000 0000000000 0000000000 00000000	0000000000 0000000000 000	0000000000 0000000000 0000000000 000	0000000000 0000000000 00000000
Favor moderately	0000000000 000000	0000000000 0000000000 0000000000 000000000	0000000000 0000000000 000000000	0000000000 0000000000 00	0000000000 0000000000 0000000000 000	0000000000 0000000000 0000
Not sure	0000000000 0000	0000000000 00000	0000000000 0	000000000	0000000000 0000000000 00	0000000000 0000000
Oppose moderately	000000000		0000	0000		0000000000 0
Oppose strongly	00000	0000000000 00000	0000000000 00000000	0000000000 0000000000 0000000000 0000	0000000000 00	0000000000 0000000000

Note: Each 0 = 1 percent.

Source: Constructed by the author.

FIGURE 5.10

Attitudes of General Public, by Education, toward a City Policy of Making Abortion Available to Teenagers, Southern City, 1977

PERCENTAGE

	Less Than High School (N = 29)	High School (N = 60)	College (N = 87)	Graduate Education (N = 39)
Favor strongly	0000000000 0000000000 0000000000	0000000000 0000000000 0000000000 0	0000000000 0000000000 0000000000 000000	0000000000 0000000000 0000000000 0000000000 000000000
Favor moderately	0000000000 0000	0000000000 0000000000 00	0000000000 0000000000 0000000000 0000	0000000000 0000000000 0000
Not sure	0000000	0000000000 0000000	0000000000 00000000	00000000
Oppose moderately	0000000000 0000	00000	000	00000000
Oppose strongly	0000000000 0000000000 0000000000 00000	0000000000 0000000000 00000	0000000000	0000000000 0

Note: Each 0 = 1 percent.

Source: Constructed by the author.

115

FIGURE 5.11

Attitudes of General Public, by Religion, toward a Policy of Making Abortion Available to Teenagers, Farmville, 1977

	Conservative Protestant (N = 28)	Mainline Protestant (N = 155)	Roman Catholic (N = 7)	Other (N = 35)
Favor strongly		0000000000 0000000000 0	0000000000 0000	00000000
Favor moderately	000	0000000000 000000000		0000000000 0000000000 000000000
Not sure	0000000000 0000000000 0000000	0000000000 0	0000000000 0000000000 000000000	0000000000 0000000000 000
Oppose moderately	0000000000 00	0000000000 0000		0000000000 0000
Oppose strongly	0000000000 0000000000 0000000000 0000000000 0000000000 00000000	0000000000 0000000000 0000000000 00000	0000000000 0000000000 0000000000 0000000000 0000000000 0000000	0000000000 0000000000 000000

PERCENTAGE

Note: Each 0 = 1 percent.

Source: Constructed by the author.

dren, religion, education, race, occupation, and income. Of these
many demographic characteristics only two were statistically significant in the general public in Southern City: education and occupation.
Service workers, clerical workers, and unemployed persons were
the most likely social groups to be opposed to providing abortions for
teenagers (see Figure 5.9). Education correlated clearly with the
degree of opposition to abortions for teenagers. Those with less than
high school education were the most likely to oppose abortion for teenagers, while those with college or graduate education were the most
likely to favor a policy of providing abortion to teenagers (see Figure
5.10). Age, sex, race, religion, number of children, and income
were not predictors of opposition or support for abortion for teenagers.
A fairly homogeneous community attitude favoring abortion for teenagers existed in Southern City.

In Farmville the only demographic factor predictive of attitude
toward abortion for teenagers was religion (Figure 5.11). As might
be expected, the Roman Catholics in the sample and the conservative
Protestants were opposed to abortion for teenagers more than half of
the time. However, mainline Protestants (Methodists, Presbyterians,
Episcopalians) were not far behind the level of opposition to the policy
voiced by the Roman Catholics and the conservative Protestants. For
example, at the end of the continuum of favorability toward the policy,
Roman Catholics were favorable by a four to one margin over the conservative Protestants.

The teenage mothers were a special situation. It is important
to remember that they were the teenage women in both communities
who in 1976 chose to have a baby rather than to seek an abortion;
hence a strong belief that abortion for teenagers is undesirable is not
surprising. Even so, more than half of the teenage mothers who did
not choose abortion for themselves, usually on strongly held grounds,
either favored a community policy of abortion for teenagers or were
neutral toward it.

LOCAL, STATE, AND NATIONAL
ACCEPTANCE OF ABORTION

Positions taken by state judges, state legislators, state human
services administrators, congressmen, and the U.S. Department of
Health, Education and Welfare on the issue of abortions for teenagers
appear in Figure 5.12. The pattern of service providers at the local
level favoring provision of abortion to teenagers more than any other
group held true at both the state and national levels. A larger percentage of state human services administrators (61 percent) strongly
favored this policy than any other group in the entire study. There

FIGURE 5.12

State and Federal Decision Makers' Attitudes toward a Policy of Allowing Abortions for Teenagers, 1977

PERCENTAGE

	North Carolina Judges (N = 125)	North Carolina Legislators (N = 101)	North Carolina HSAs (N = 58)	U.S. Congressmen (N = 83)	HEW* (N = 43)
Favor strongly	0000000000 0000000000 0000000000 000000	0000000000 0000000000 0000000000	0000000000 0000000000 0000000000 0000000000 0000000000 0000000000 0	0000000000 0000000000 0000000000	0000000000 0000000000 0000000000 0000000000 0000000000 0000000000
Favor moderately	0000000000 0000000000 0000000000 0	0000000000 0000000000 0000000000 0000	0000000000 0000000000 00000	0000000000 00000000	0000000000 0000000000 0000000000
Not sure	0000000000 00	0000000000	0000000000	0000000000 0	00
Oppose moderately	0000000000	0000000000 000	00	0000000000 000	00000
Oppose strongly	0000000000 0	0000000000 000	00	0000000000 0000000000 00000000	00000

*HEW = Department of Health, Education and Welfare human services administrators.

Note: Each 0 = 1 percent.

Source: Constructed by the author.

was a remarkable similarity of attitudes among Southern City policy makers, service providers, and state and national human services administrators: they all strongly favored a policy of providing abortion to teenagers. State judges and state legislators were less favorable toward the policy, but less than 20 percent opposed the idea of communities having policies favoring abortion for teenagers. At the state and national level only the U.S. senators and representatives registered significantly increased opposition to abortion for teenagers. Of the congressmen who responded, 40 percent opposed a policy of abortion for teenagers. It is not possible to tell to what extent the responding congressmen are representative of the U.S. Congress as a whole.

Policy makers—whether local board members in Farmville or Southern City or state judges, state legislators, or national congressmen—tended to be generally comparable in their degree of acceptance of a policy of abortion for teenagers. Comparatively speaking, the service providers at the local, state, and national levels were all consistently more favorable than the policy makers toward a policy of abortion for teenagers.

ABORTION WITHOUT PARENTAL CONSENT

Parental consent is one of the more inflammatory policy issues in the area of birth control, especially in regard to providing abortion without parental consent. We phrased question 17 to test for a policy of "allowing abortion for teenagers without parental consent, if necessary." The addition of the phrase "if necessasy" allowed each respondent to define whatever conditions might necessitate abortion without parents' having to give consent. One respondent might imagine a situation in which the parents refuse to give consent in face of a situation in which the girl faces possible death or a very high probability of the birth of a deformed infant. Other respondents might imagine circumstances in which the teenage girl simply "prefers" not to tell her parents for her own convenience. The results show that for whatever reason, dire or seemingly inconsequential, the effect of adding a provision of "abortion without parental consent, if necessary" had the effect of significantly reducing support for the policy of abortion for teenagers among nearly all the groups studied except the teenagers themselves.

Significant Increases in Opposition

In Farmville two-thirds of the policy makers and half of the service providers opposed provision of abortion to teenagers without requiring parental consent. Seventy percent of the general public were in opposition, as were half of the teen mothers. Abortion without parental consent did not have majority support among any Farmville group.

Adding a qualification about parental consent reduced support for abortion for teenagers among all groups in Southern City. Nevertheless, a majority (two-thirds) of the policy makers were still either positive or neutral, 79 percent of the service providers were either positive or neutral, and 53 percent of the general public supported abortion for teenagers even without parental consent. It made very little difference to the teenage mothers whether the abortion policy required or did not require parental consent.

Another way to calculate the impact of adding the condition that abortion be made available without requiring parental consent is to calculate the increase in opposition generated by adding that condition. The percentage increase in the "oppose moderately" and "oppose strongly" categories created by adding the proviso that parental consent not be required is shown:

Policy Makers		Service Providers		General Public		Teenage Mothers	
F	SC	F	SC	F	SC	F	SC
113	280	512	600	40	95	16	8

A Political Explanation

A political explanation may be the most reasonable one for the figures above. The group most directly vulnerable to criticism or lawsuit is the service providers; hence, they exhibited a large increase in opposition to the idea of not requiring parental consent. The next most vulnerable group is the elected and appointed policy makers, who must answer for their concepts of voter opinion on the policy idea of allowing abortion to teenagers without parental consent. The teenagers seemed to wonder whether there is an issue here at all. Their views on the acceptability of abortion for teenagers was virtually unaffected by adding the idea of not requiring parental consent. What is curious is that all of these opinions appear within a political milieu in which the U.S. Supreme Court has made abortion without requiring parental consent the law of the land. As if often the case, however, the Supreme Court is in an "out front" leadership role and has set a standard for the nation, which typically will slowly conform its thinking and acceptance. The current antiabortion movement in the United States may lead to a different outcome.

A Parental Authority Explanation

There is a general assumption prevalent that parents do not want to give up their prerogative of controlling the medical care given to their teenage daughters, especially in the area of contraceptives and abortion. Public opposition to abortion when parental consent is not required increased by 20 percent in Farmville and by 23 percent in Southern City.

Support for Abortion without Parental Consent

Who favored abortion for teenagers in Farmville without requiring parental consent? Support came from members of the general public who are younger (see Figure 5.13), who are professionals (see Figures 5.14 and 5.15), and who have not yet had children (see Figure 5.16). Conversely, the opposition to a policy of allowing abortion to teenagers without parental consent became more intense with increasing age. The percentage of persons in the "strongly opposed" category shows a steady progression by age from the twenties (40 percent opposition), to the thirties (54 percent), forties (57 percent), fifties (67 percent), and finally to those in their sixties and older (75 percent). Even so, the attitudes of the Farmville general public remained remarkably homogeneous with regard to sex, marital status, church membership, education, race, and income.

Influences of Income and Occupation

In Southern City the only demographic characteristics that produced significant differences in attitude toward allowing teenagers to obtain abortions without parental consent were income and occupation. These differences were only marginally significant (0.04 and 0.03 levels, respectively).

Opposition and Political Exposure

Increase in opposition to permitting abortions for teenagers with the proviso that parental consent not be required was greatest among state human services administrators (350 percent). These persons are the most directly accountable to the courts and legislators for policy decisions having possible legal implications or creating public displeasure. The judges in the state of North Carolina showed a considerably stronger opposition to abortion for teenagers without parental

FIGURE 5.13

Attitudes of General Public, by Age, toward a Policy of Allowing Abortion for Teenagers without Parental Consent, if Necessary, Farmville, 1977

	Aged 20 to 30 (N = 47)	Aged 30 to 40 (N = 44)	Aged 40 to 50 (N = 59)	Aged 50 to 60 (N = 51)	Aged 60 and Over (N = 24)
Favor strongly	0000000000 00000	00000	0000000000 0	00000000	
Favor moderately	0000000000 000000000	0000000000 000000	0000	00000000	0000
Not sure	0000000000 000	000000000	0000000000 000000	000000	0000000000 000
Oppose moderately	0000000000 000	0000000000 000000	0000000000 00	0000000000 0	00000000
Oppose strongly	0000000000 0000000000 0000000000 0000000000	0000000000 0000000000 0000000000 0000000000 0000	0000000000 0000000000 0000000000 0000000000 0000000	0000000000 0000000000 0000000000 0000000000 0000000	0000000000 0000000000 0000000000 0000000000 0000000000 0000000000 00000

Note: Each 0 = 1 percent.

Source: Constructed by the author.

FIGURE 5.14

Attitudes of General Public, by Occupation, toward a Policy of Allowing Abortion for Teenagers without Parental Consent, if Necessary, Farmville, 1977

PERCENTAGE

	Profes-sional (N = 36)	Mana-gerial (N = 56)	Clerical (N = 34)	Service (N = 19)	Blue Collar (N = 33)	Unem-ployed (N = 57)	Other (N = 2)
Favor strongly	0000000000 000000	0000	0000000000 00		000000000	0000000	
Favor moderately	0000000000 0000000000 0000000000 0	0000000	0000000000 000	0000000000 00	000000	0000	
Not sure	00000000	0000000000 0	000000	0000000000 00	000000000	0000000000 0000000000	
Oppose moderately	000000	0000000000 00000	0000000000 000000000	0000000000 00	0000000000 00	000000000	
Oppose strongly	0000000000 0000000000 0000000000 000000000	0000000000 0000000000 0000000000 0000000000 0000000000 0000000000 000	0000000000 0000000000 0000000000 0000000000	0000000000 0000000000 0000000000 0000000000 0000000000 0000000000 0000	0000000000 0000000000 0000000000 0000000000 0000000000 0000000000 0000	0000000000 0000000000 0000000000 0000000000 0000000000 0000000000	0000000000 0000000000 0000000000 0000000000 0000000000 0000000000 0000000000 0000000000 0000000000 0000000000 0000000000

Note: Each 0 = 1 percent.

Source: Constructed by the author.

123

FIGURE 5.15

Attitudes of General Public, by Occupation, toward a Policy of Allowing Abortion for Teenagers without Parental Consent, if Necessary, Southern City, 1977

PERCENTAGE

	Professional (N = 45)	Managerial (N = 42)	Clerical (N = 28)	Service (N = 23)	Blue Collar (N = 9)	Unemployed (N = 68)
Favor strongly	0000000000 00000000	000000	0000000000 0000000	0000000000 0000000000 0000000	0000000000 00	0000000000 0000
Favor moderately	0000000000 0000000000 0000000000 0000000000	0000000000 0000000000 0000000000	0000000000 0000000000 00000	0000	0000000000 0000000000 0000000000 000	0000000000 000000
Not sure	0000000000 00000000	0000000000 00000	0000000000 0	0000	0000000000 0000000000 00	0000000000 00000
Oppose moderately	0000000000 000	0000000000 0000000000 00000	0000000000 0	0000000000 0000000	0000000000 0000000000 00	0000000000 000
Oppose strongly	0000000000 0	0000000000 0000000000 00000	0000000000 0000000000 000000	0000000000 0000000000 0000000000 00000000	0000000000 0	0000000000 0000000000 0000000000 00

Note: Each 0 = 1 percent.

Source: Constructed by the author.

FIGURE 5.16

Attitudes of General Public, by Number of Children, toward a Policy of Allowing Abortion for Teenagers without Parental Consent, it Necessary, Farmville, 1977

PERCENTAGE

	No Children (N = 47)	1 or 2 Children (N = 114)	3 or More Children (N = 76)
Favor strongly	0000000000 000000000	00000000	0000
Favor moderately	0000000000 0000000	0000000000 0	0000
Not sure	0000000000 0	0000000000 00	0000000000 000
Oppose moderately	00	0000000000 000	0000000000 000000
Oppose strongly	0000000000 0000000000 0000000000 0000000000 0000000000 0	0000000000 0000000000 0000000000 0000000000 0000000000 000000	0000000000 0000000000 0000000000 0000000000 0000000000 0000000000 000

Note: Each 0 = 1 percent.

Source: Constructed by the author.

125

consent, increasing their opposition by 150 percent. State legislators, however, showed less concern about adding permission for abortion without parental consent, while national congressmen and federal human services providers showed the least concern about any consequences of additional public disapproval if parental consent were not required.

Support

Large value gaps exist between the policies for care supported by the APHA and some of the groups included in this study. Clearly the service providers on all levels were the most supportive of providing abortions for teenagers (see Figures 5.8 and 5.12). Less support existed among the policy makers, especially in Farmville and the U.S. Congress. Only one-third of the general public in Farmville and two-thirds of the general public in Southern City supported abortion for teenagers. When the proviso was added that abortion be available without parental consent, general public support in Farmville dwindled to 20 percent. In Southern City the level of support fell to 40 percent. Support of abortion for teenagers decreased among all state and national groups when abortion without parental consent was proposed as a policy. On simply the issue of making abortion available to teenagers, a clear majority of state judges and legislators, as well as nearly all of the human services administrators at the state and federal level, were supportive. Adding the requirement that teenagers be able to get abortions without parental consent significantly reduced the level of support among state human services administrators and state judges. Even so, about half of the state legislators in North Carolina, and half of the congressmen who responded, were supportive of a policy to allow teenagers to obtain abortions without parental consent. Eighty percent of the state and federal human services administrators still supported the policy of abortion for teenagers even when the condition of "without parental consent" was added. Abortion for teenagers is a value on which there was a consensus among at least a majority of all the respondents. Abortion for teenagers without parental consent was a much more divisive issue.

Persistent Failure to Manage Fertility

It is important for teenagers to be able to control their fertility. Some teenagers in Farmville and in Southern City are successfully managing their fertility, but large numbers are not. We have documented wide-ranging value differences among the two communities and the state and national administrators and policy makers. If, in spite of the value differences among adults, the teenagers in these two communities were successfully managing their fertility, the existence and persistence of these value differences might be a situation that society could affort to permit. In Chapter 6 we present our estimate and that of the National Center for Disease Control of the extent of failure among the teenagers in these two communities to manage their sexuality successfully.

6

TEEN ACCESS TO CONTRACEPTIVES

There is no real program organized that specifically
makes a point to offer family planning advice or services to teenagers. Doctors usually do it with the knowledge of the parents. Usually the child's mother or older
sister gets pills from the M.D. or the Health Department
and gives them to the teenager. But the Health Department regulations make this difficult. It's a folk solution
that the Health Department makes it hard to carry out.

A concerned Farmville physician

On the basis of current levels of sexual activity among teenagers
in surveys across the United States, 661 of the 3,074 teenage women
in Farmville and 5,647 of the 26,260 teenage women in Southern City
were sexually active in 1976.* Opinions range from active condem-
nation of the current levels of sexual activity among teenagers to feelings that teenage sexual activity is not necessarily bad in itself. But
certainly, in our opinion, teen behavior has yet to become sexually
responsible. In this chapter we focus on programs in the two communities that attempt to provide contraceptive help to sexually active
teenagers.

---

*According to the Alan Guttmacher Institute (1976) the percent-
ages of teenagers who were estimated to be sexually active in 1974/75
are as follows: age 13, 14 percent; age 14, 17 percent; age 15, 24
percent; age 16, 31 percent; age 17, 35 percent; age 18, 43 percent;
and age 19, 51 percent. The 1976 estimates for Farmville and Southern City are probably conservative, inasmuch as the level of sexual
activity has been rising every year in the 1970s.

SUMMARY OVERVIEW

Policy makers, service providers, and the general public in both communities were asked what local programs offer contraceptive services to young teenagers. As might be expected, the information levels among the policy makers and service providers were considerably higher than among the general public. Farmville policy makers viewed the local Health Department as the primary source (38 percent of the time), with local private physicians as the second most important source. (See Table 6.1.) One-fourth of the policy makers said either that they did not know what programs offered services or that they felt no local program offered contraceptives to younger teenagers. Service providers responded similarly, but with increased emphasis on the Public Health Department and local physicians as sources of

TABLE 6.1

What Local Programs Offer Contraceptive Services to Young Teenagers: Views of Policy Makers, Service Providers, and General Public, Farmville and Southern City, 1977
(percent)

Contraceptive Services	Policy Makers		Service Providers		General Public	
	F	SC	F	SC	F	SC
None available	8	0	4	2	33	19
Public Health Department	38	49	54	47	49	0
Private physician	22	11	36	16	9	3
Department of Social Services	8	0	2	0	3	5
Schools	2	0	2	0	0	0
Gas stations	10	0	2	0	0	0
Hospital	1	15	0	8	0	7
Clinics	0	10	0	10	0	11
Other	22	0	8	0	8	0
Total response excluding don't know	59	0	52	0	91	0
Don't know (number)	7	12	4	0	139	122
Total response (number)	66	57	56	55	230	220
Individuals (number)	43	40	38	35	210	215

Note: F = Farmville; SC = Southern City.

Source: Compiled by the author.

contraceptives for young teenagers. Among the general public 60 percent said they did not know of any program offering contraceptives to younger teenagers, and of the 40 percent who did say they knew, one-third said there was no program available, leaving about one-quarter of the general public who felt they knew of a program offering contraceptives to younger teenagers. The service providers ranked private physicians as a major source only slightly less important than the Health Department. Policy makers and the general public viewed the private physician's role as less important. Farmville teenagers in the general public sample who responded said teenagers go to the Public Health Department (60 percent of the time) or outside the area (20 percent of the time), or said no services were available (20 percent of the time).

CONSISTENT DIFFERENCES BETWEEN COMMUNITIES

Continuing a now consistent difference between the two communities, Southern City respondents named several more sources of contraceptive help for younger teenagers. (See Table 6.1.) In addition to the Public Health Department, they mentioned local hospitals and clinics, two sources not available in Farmville. Policy makers and service providers viewed the Health Department and private physicians as the main sources. The adult general public also named the Health Department, hospitals, and clinics as major sources, but evidently felt that private physicians were not a source, naming them only 3 percent of the time. On the other hand, since the question was phrased to ask respondents to identify programs, this nearly nonmention of private physicians may be appropriate.

Service providers, policy makers, and the general public in Southern City were much less likely to say no services were available, but 60 percent of respondents in the general public in both communities did say they did not know. As in the cases of abortion and counseling, a wider range of options was reported available to teenagers in Southern City, which teen respondents confirmed. One interesting note is that both service providers and policy makers in Farmville mentioned gas stations as a source. While this stretches the concept of a program, it is significant that machines vending condoms in gas stations were thought of as an apparently important source of contraceptive assistance for local teenagers. No one in Southern City mentioned gas stations.

CONTRACEPTIVE SERVICES FOR YOUNGER TEENAGERS

Farmville Policy Makers

> Public health, mental health, and the Department of Social
> Services work awfully close together—it's kind of a puzzle
> they fit together. They are awfully good about referral.
> We're a small county but we're close. Any time someone
> has a problem, it's found out and we refer them on where
> to go to.
>
> A Farmville commissioner

> I did try to go to the health clinic 'cause we didn't have
> any insurance or anything. They told me to go see so-
> cial services. They said we made too much money—
> about $100 more than you need to get in. For a while I
> didn't know what I was going to do.
>
> A pregnant 17-year-old
Farmville girl

Are the elected county commissioners and city councilmen in
Farmville aware of programs that offer actual contraceptive services
to Farmville teenagers? Not really. Of the ten interviewed, two
said they simply did not know; one said none existed; four mentioned
the Health Department; one mentioned private physicians, one mentioned service stations; and one said he did not know, but he assumed
that "mental health and the Health Department and school psycholo-
gists offer birth control. I'm sure the school system has adviser
services." The Farmville commissioner quoted above waxed eloquent
about the close working relationship of the various departments. The
reader will be able to judge to what extent this commissioner's strong
confidence is warranted when responses from the service providers
to which he referred are discussed below.

Of the named influentials interviewed, half mentioned the Health
Department and half said they did not know of any services in Farmville.

None of the three social services board members or the health
board members interviewed knew of any services available to young
teenagers in Farmville. One mental health board member saw "gas
stations, drugstores, and females" as the main programmatic sources
of such birth control assistance. Two felt that "some docs" might
offer help. Two thought perhaps the Health Department might, but
were not sure. One responded that the "Department of Social Services
has something on family planning. Should think the Health Department
would too."

The random pattern of scattered information available among board members reviewed thus far in Farmville was continued by the school board members. Two felt gas stations were the best sources of contraceptive help to teenagers in Farmville. Of the eight board members, one thought of the local Health Department, but dismissed it as an important source in belief that it probably required parental consent. One said he had been told that some doctors would give birth control help to Farmville teenagers. Two said the local doctors were the "only" source. One looked up the name of a local obstetrician in the telephone book and gave that name. The last school board member interviewed said no birth control help was available in the county.

The randomness of information exhibited by these key policy-making board members is impressive because it was so consistent from board to board and member to member. The lack of information among key policy makers in the community also had important implications for the availability of services to the teens themselves. If the people responsible for making and overseeing decisions to offer services were unaware of programs, one could only expect the teens to be substantially less informed. This was, in fact, largely the picture given by the teen respondents.

The idea that gas stations were the best source of contraceptive services for Farmville teenagers harks back to several years ago, when some local gas stations offered low-quality but high-priced condoms in their men's rooms, a practice not currently followed by any of the stations visited by researchers.

Southern City Policy Makers

Elected commissioners and board members in Southern City exhibited a curious mixture of information levels, not unlike those of board members and commissioners in Farmville. One difference in the response pattern, however, was for Southern City officials either to name the Health Department or not to know of any sources of services.

The three commissioners we interviewed ran the gamut of information levels. One said no services were available to Southern City teenagers. One had heard that the Health Department was a good source. The third named the Health Department, then added explanatory details: "All who have abortions or deliveries receive birth control counseling and follow-up services." Three health board members mentioned the Health Department as a source. Both mental health board members who participated in the study named the Health Department and private physicians. Only one of the five mental health board members knew the Health Department offered services to younger teenagers. Half of the ten Southern City school board members knew of no sources of services. The other five all mentioned the Health Department, three of them also naming a local abortion clinic.

The opposite of what we had expected was turning out to be the case. We had predicted that information about abortion would be less prevalent than information about family planning services among the policy makers of the two communities. Instead, the pattern developed for policy makers to be rather well informed about the sources of abortion services for teenagers, but relatively less informed about sources of contraceptive care for teenagers. Admittedly, abortion is more dramatic than preventing unwanted conceptions. What impressed us is that there was far more consistent information available among policy makers about temporary cures (abortions) for teenagers' failures to manage their fertility successfully than about programs helping teenagers prevent unwanted pregnancies in the first place.

Farmville Service Providers

Physicians

Among seven Farmville physicians we interviewed, all of them said the private physicians of Farmville prescribed contraceptives. It was not clear whether these physicians would dispense contraceptives to girls under 18 without the signature of a parent. A head nurse at the local hospital mentioned the Health Department, but added that it helped "only after delivery" of a child.

Social Workers

Social workers were well informed. All but one of the Social Services Department staff mentioned both the Health Department and local physicians. Among the four mental health staff members interviewed, one said the Health Department offered contraceptives, but only "with parental consent." Two other staff members said they did not know. Another mental health staff member identified as working with teenagers said she was "not that familiar with the resources, but I assume that medical doctors of the Health Department do."

Pharmacists

When asked what programs offer actual contraceptive services in Farmville, one of the pharmacists replied: "The school went into oral sex in their discussion, but did not go into details of [contraceptive] supplies." Among the other pharmacists in Farmville, two said the Health Department supplied pills; one did not know; and two said there were no birth control services available to teenagers in the community.

School Personnel

Farmville school administrators seemed relatively well informed: over half of the 11 mentioned the Health Department; 2 mentioned family doctors; and only 2 said they did not know.

Among the four Farmville school counselors identified as counseling teenagers, three said they did not know if there was a source for birth control services in the community. The fourth said the "Health Department provides information—but I do not think it is an actual program—just available service."

Service providers in Farmville seemed somewhat better informed than the policy makers, but they differed among themselves over whether any actual program offered contraceptive assistance to sexually active Farmville teenagers. This ambivalence was reflected in responses of the teenage mothers. Some of them were able to get contraceptives without parents' permission at an age of less than 18; some of them tried and were refused; some of them believed they could get contraceptives only by taking their mothers with them; and some of them knew that the Health Department never checked to see if the person they brought was really their mother. Clearly there was no consistent message for teens who were in need of service.

Southern City Service Providers

Physicians

All of the 14 Southern City medical doctors who participated in the study mentioned the Health Department as a source for birth control services to teenagers. Most of them also mentioned private physicians as sources of family planning services.

Other Service Providers

Six of the seven Department of Social Services staff members who participated mentioned the Health Department as the best source. All mental health service providers interviewed mentioned the Health Department. Of the five participating pharmacists, three knew of no services available to Southern City teenagers; one mentioned a non-existent Planned Parenthood clinic; and one knew of the Health Department clinic. Among Southern City school administrators, four knew of no contraceptive help for teenagers and seven mentioned the Health Department. Of the three school counselors interviewed, two knew of the Health Department, and one knew of no sources of contraceptive help for sexually active Southern City teenagers.

Service Providers' Pattern

It appears that in Southern City the service providers—the physicians, social services workers, mental health staff, school administrators, and counselors—were generally well informed about the availability of contraceptive services for teenagers at the local Health Department. A definite pattern seemed to be emerging from the service providers' answers in the two communities: far more service providers, as well as policy makers, knew of abortion services than of birth control services. What came as a constant surprise to us was that, like the policy makers, the service providers who did not know of the availability of birth control services at the Health Department did seem to know consistently of the abortion services (or service referrals) available at the Health Department. Thus, abortion, the short-term cure for teenagers' failures to manage their fertility, is better known than the preventive services offered by the Health Department, by clinics, and by the private physicians.

When the lessened level of information among policy makers and even service providers about birth control services, compared with abortion services, is taken into account, it is not surprising that not more than one-fourth of the general public knew of any birth control services available to teenagers in either community.

THE FARMVILLE BIRTH CONTROL PROGRAM

> There's entirely too many of them getting pregnant with the services we have if they had the motivation to get some type of birth control. The thing is, so many of them don't want their parents to know.
>
> A Farmville Health Department family planning staff member

Physicians

For teenagers 18 and younger, the search for birth control help in Farmville was a task requiring persistence and parental consent in the private sector and promiscuity in the public sector. It was not possible to get the cooperation of all the Farmville physicians in our attempt to determine the number of Farmville teenagers receiving birth control help from their private physicians. We were able to obtain specific information from only three physicians offering birth control assistance to teenagers 18 and younger.

One of the physicians said he had seen about 24 birth control patients aged 18 or younger in 1976; 20 of these young women were on the pill. A second physician said he had provided birth control methods to 50 young women aged 18 and younger during 1976; 35 of these were on the pill and 15 were wearing IUDs.

The third physician, who was considered the most actively involved physician providing birth control to teenagers, said that all the general practitioners did family planning and prescribed the pill or the IUD. He asserted that we would come up with a number "close to zero" of 13-, 14-, and 15-year-olds in Farmville who were obtaining contraceptives without parental consent. He conjectured that maybe a "few 16-year-olds" might be getting contraceptives without parental consent; but, he reasserted, "Few 13-, 14-, and 15-year-olds can get birth control with or without parental consent." Thus, while most Farmville physicians did offer birth control assistance to teenagers, it was seldom without parental consent; and teenagers were actually getting birth control services, in the opinion of the physician quoted above.

Public Health Department

Parental consent was required by the physician directing the public health clinic. However, he made exceptions for "promiscuous" teenagers. He declared a teenager "promiscuous," and thus eligible for birth control assistance without parental consent, if she (1) had had an abortion, (2) had had a child, or (3) had venereal disease.

For the sexually active Farmville teenager who sought birth control services from the Public Health Department, whether she qualified as promiscuous or not, the procedure was much the same as for obtaining a pregnancy test. She must call for an appointment, go to social services for certification of eligibility for Title 19 or Title 20 funds, and bring verification of her parents' income to social services. Then she went to the Health Department clinic accompanied by an adult female, presumed to be her mother, who, witnessed by authorized Health Department personnel, signed a permission slip for the girl to be given birth control help.

The Farmville family planning program got its start about 1961, when two local doctors grew weary of the number of low-income deliveries burdening their private practices. They suggested it would be beneficial if the Health Department would see the low-income patients. In 1966 the Department of Social Services made money available to the Health Department to pay for birth control services to its clients. In 1968 the state began giving federal family planning funds to the program. The Health Department policy had been to participate in all available state and federal funding programs. The program in 1976 was essentially a state-funded program with additional funds coming from collection of Title 19 and Title 20 fees by the Department of Social Services.

Third-Party Reimbursement

The $53 per patient paid for the initial visit under Department of Social Services certification seems a powerful attraction for the funding needs of the Farmville program. As the director of the Health Department family planning clinic observed in our interview with him, the local county commissioners provide 65 percent of the funds for the Health Department, and "in a small county it is hard to ask commissioners to pay that much money." At the time of this comment, the director was talking about the infeasibility of the Health Department's offering pregnancy tests "willy-nilly" to anyone who wanted to know if she was pregnant. It had been the policy of the family planning program personnel in Farmville to operate the program within established organizational guidelines. Thus, in the matter of funding, the Health Department had always sought and received maximum state and federal funding, believing that without federal and state funds the program would not be feasible.

The official leaflet distributed to the public proclaimed that the Monday clinics offering family planning were for and available to "everyone." In practice the department had been careful to stay within official guidelines, which, while also claiming to provide family planning for "everyone," in reality had been focused on the low-income women eligible for social services. Thus, the Health Department asked all potential clients to obtain social services certification of eligibility (following nationally recognized guidelines). When asked what requiring social services' certification does to potential clients' feelings, a Health Department staff member replied, "Some get agitated and say, 'I'll go to my doctor.'" As the director of the family planning program said, "We encourage them to use their own physician."

Social Services Screening

What, in practice, was the impact of the social services' screening requirement? Health Department personnel reported two different effects. Once, concerned about the effect of requiring that screening, the Health Department staff asked 20 potential patients if they objected to being required to go to social services first for certification. Only two said they objected.

One of the professional staff of the family planning clinic reported on the impact of the social services certification requirement. In February 1977, 80 Farmville residents seeking family planning services were screened by the Department of Social Services, and in March 1977, 70 were screened. Of the 150 persons screened over the two-month period, only 28 were declared eligible. Thus, 72 percent of the Farmville residents who sought family planning services during the two months were declared ineligible for the Public Health Department program.

It appears that messages at several levels were being communicated to Farmville women seeking family planning services at the public health clinic. If the public was confused by the several levels of messages, it was because clinic staff members were in fact giving several messages. As one staff member said, "We send 35 to 40 people for Title 20 certification every week. Our program is open to anyone who just asks. We have a lot [of Farmville residents] that resent it [being sent to social services]. We lose some, but most of them can afford to pay anyway. They [the Department of Social Services] have worked very good with us." By working "good with us" the staff member meant the practice of a social worker's coming to the Health Department to interview potential family planning candidates for social services certification.

When we interviewed the clinic director, he said that the practice was working very well. The clinic staff said the social worker had, unknown to the clinic director, stopped coming to the Health Department some months earlier. The social worker did not like the fact that there was no place to interview a prospective patient except in the public waiting room, and also disliked the inconvenience of being separated from her files. The opinion of one staff member seemed to be that it was just as well that the Department of Social Services screened out as much as 72 percent of Farmville residents seeking family planning services from the Health Department clinic, because "We usually turn down enough one clinic day to fill up the next." One of the professional staff observed that since the current physician-in-charge had come, the number of patients served had dropped from "50 to 60" per Monday to 15.

Table 4.3 summarizes the Farmville family planning program's activities from January through December 1976. It shows that 931 persons received family planning services during that year. Since 264 files were closed that year, the number of residents actually receiving contraceptive services was 667. As is indicated under "medical services," nearly all of these 667 persons received a breast exam, heart and lung exam, pelvic exam, pap smear, gonorrhea test, blood test, urinalysis, blood pressure test, other lab tests, and "other medical exams." Of the 648 persons in the program using contra-

TABLE 6.2

Selected Vital Statistics, Farmville, 1976

Item	Total	White	Nonwhite
Population			
Total	33,183	25,898	7,285
Males	15,781	12,396	3,385
Females	17,402	13,502	3,900
Natural increase	214	115	99
Live Births			
Total	538	369	169
Males	262	179	83
Females	276	190	86
Attendant			
Physician in hospital	537	369	168
Physician not in hospital	1	0	1
Midwife or other	0	0	0
Premature births	50	24	26
Out-of-wedlock	99	21	78
Fetal and infant mortality			
Perinatal deaths	15	9	6
Fetal deaths	6	4	2
Attendant			
Physician in hospital	6	4	2
Physician not in hospital	0	0	0
Midwife and other	0	0	0
Out-of-wedlock	2	0	2
Neonatal (under 28 days)	9	5	4
Postneonatal (28 days to 1 year)	2	0	2
Infant deaths (under 1 year)	11	5	6

Source: North Carolina Vital Statistics, Division of Health Services, Administrative Services Section, Public Health Statistics Branch, 1976.

FIGURE 6.1

Percentage of Females Aged 13 to 17 and 18 to 19 Served by Public
Family Planning Program, Farmville, 1976

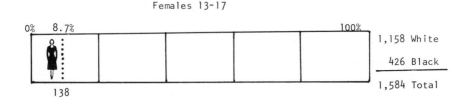

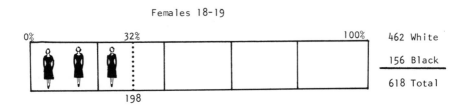

Source: Constructed by the author.

ceptives, 598 (92 percent) were using the pill, 29 (5 percent) were
using the IUD, 1 was using the diaphragm, 6 were using foam, and
19 were using nothing. Table 6.2 gives selected data for 1976 for
Farmville, including live births and fetal and infant mortality.

According to the state family planning program, in 1976 the
Farmville family planning program served 138 people, or 8.7 percent
of the female population aged 13 to 17 and 198 people or 32 percent of
women aged 18 to 19 (see Figure 6.1). Table 4.3 shows 37 Medicaid-
reimbursable initial and annual medical visits in 1976 along with 158
Title 20-reimbursable initial and annual medical visits. Thus, out of
611 new and continuing patients in 1976, 195 (32 percent) were Medi-
caid- or Title 20-reimbursable. It appears that perhaps two-thirds
of the family planning patients were not certified as eligible for reim-
bursement to the Health Department clinic.

THE SOUTHERN CITY BIRTH CONTROL PROGRAM

Teenagers under 18

For teenagers under 18 the search for birth control help in
Southern City usually led to the Health Department family planning

program. The program operated not only in the Health Department itself but also in a nearby large hospital and in four satellite community outposts that offered seven clinics a week. Statistics for 1976/77 indicate that 71 percent of new patients (1,304) attended the Health Department clinic, 18 percent (343) started at the hospital clinic, and the remaining 11 percent (199) were distributed among the satellite clinics —5 percent (64) at one and 2 percent each at the other three (an average of 45 women per clinic).

The main family planning clinic in the Health Department operated all day on Thursdays, seeing both continuing and new patients; every Tuesday from 5:45 P.M., with late evening clinics on the second and fourth Tuesdays and the first, third, and fourth Wednesdays; and every Saturday morning from 8:30 to about 11:00. Of the 7,276 active patients in the program during 1976, approximately 22 percent were teenagers.

Clinic Procedures

To obtain help with birth control, a teenager had only to present herself at one of the clinics, where she was assigned to a counselor with whom she could discuss her needs. If she only wanted a contraceptive, she went through the clinic and was provided whatever method she chose. Under only two circumstances must an individual under 18 obtain parental consent: when she wanted to have an IUD inserted or when she wanted county funds to pay for an abortion. Under all other circumstances the family planning services were available to all sexually active individuals without regard to age or ability to pay. One staff member reported that in 1976 the median income of family planning recipients in the program was about $10,000 per year. It was Health Department policy not to ask for Medicaid or Title 20 funds, because the indignity to the patient was felt to be too great a cost.

If the teenager was pregnant, she was counseled about the various alternatives available to her. The focus of the counseling was to help her think about the pregnancy in relationship to the rest of her life: her goals for a job, education, marriage, and similar concerns. If she chose to continue the pregnancy, she was enrolled in the Health Department's prenatal clinic. If she chose abortion, she was assisted in contacting one of the several abortion sources listed in Appendix E. The Health Department's criteria for choosing abortion referral sources were the availability of adequate counseling and assurance that the abortion center followed state guidelines for safe procedures. If the teenager could not pay for the abortion and asked for county abortion funds, the Health Department staff worker would, if requested, contact the teenager's parents to explain the situation and the need for parental consent in order to obtain county funds. Otherwise parents, are not contacted, except at the request of the teenager.

Types of Contraceptives

The types of contraceptives used by teenage patients are shown in Figure 6.2. What is notable about the distribution is that in contrast with the usual reliance on the pill and IUD as virtually the only two methods, about 7 percent of all patients chose foam and 8 percent,

FIGURE 6.2

Public Health Department Family Planning Program Active Clients, by Method of Birth Control, Southern City, 1976

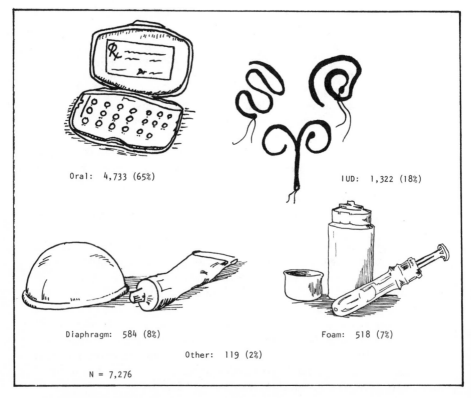

Oral: 4,733 (65%)　　　　　IUD: 1,322 (18%)

Diaphragm: 584 (8%)　　　　　Foam: 518 (7%)

Other: 119 (2%)

N = 7,276

Source: Statistics from Southern City Health Department; illustrations from Carolina Population Center.

the diaphragm. The distribution of methods chosen by teenagers was about the same as for all patients—65 percent on the pill, 18 percent using an IUD, and 17 percent using some other method.

Teenage Parity

The parity (or number of children born) of teenage participants in the Southern City Health Department family planning program appears in Table 6.3. Among teenagers under age 18 who were active in the family planning program, 63 percent had no children, 34 percent had one child, and 3 percent had two or more children. One reported having already given birth to six children.

TABLE 6.3

Public Health Department Family Planning Program Participants, by Age and Parity, Southern City, 1976

Age	Parity						
	0	1	2	3	4	5	6 and over
Under 18	409	225	17	1	1	0	1
18 to 19	530	322	78	24	4	1	1
20 to 24	1,300	983	470	168	44	11	4
25 to 29	462	530	402	210	66	37	26
30 to 34	51	95	168	146	68	44	32
35 to 39	11	22	44	38	39	18	39
40 to 44	1	3	12	10	18	10	36

Source: Southern City Health Department.

Referrals

    How did patients in the Southern City family planning program
find their way to the Health Department or one of its satellite clinics?
One of the family planning nurses at the Health Department said many
of their referrals were from private physicians. Reports from the
doctors themselves would lead one to believe this to be the case.
However, patients, when asked for their source of referral, mentioned private physicians only 1 percent of the time (see Table 6.4).
Equally surprising was the similarly minuscule number (1 percent) of
referrals credited by the patients to their social workers. It is not
possible to know the initial referring source for most of the patients
with any real precision, since 30 percent listed themselves as the referring source. It may well be that private physicians and social
workers mentioned the Health Department clinic to a patient, but her
actual coming to the clinic might have been at her own initiative. It
seems reasonable to conclude that the Health Department family planning clinic attracted new patients primarily through social contacts
with current users and through some referrals from local hospitals
and clinics. Table 6.5 presents selected data for Southern City comparable with those presented for Farmville.

TABLE 6.4

Public Health Department Family Planning Program Participants,
by Source of Referral, Southern City, 1976

Source of Referral	White	Black	Total	Percent
Self	1,163	1,012	2,175	30
Clinic	363	622	985	15
Friend	1,402	832	2,234	31
Physician	58	66	124	1
Program personnel	169	224	393	5
Advertisement	60	23	83	1
Social worker	14	26	40	1
Hospital	312	794	1,106	15
Other	77	59	136	1
Total	3,618	3,658	7,276	100

Source: Southern City Health Department.

TABLE 6.5

Selected Vital Statistics, Southern City, 1976

Item	Total	White	Nonwhite
Population			
Total	269,614	207,774	61,840
Males	132,315	102,416	29,899
Females	137,299	105,358	31,941
Natural increase	1,809	1,241	568
Live births			
Total	3,559	2,488	1,071
Males	1,860	1,309	551
Females	1,699	1,179	520
Attendant			
Physician in hospital	3,553	2,484	1,069
Physician not in hospital	4	2	2
Midwife or other	2	2	0
Premature births	288	141	147
Out–of–wedlock	539	92	447
Fetal and infant mortality			
Perinatal deaths	80	41	39
Fetal deaths	36	18	18
Attendant			
Physician in hospital	36	18	18
Physician not in hospital	0	0	0
Midwife or other	0	0	0
Out–of–wedlock	13	1	12
Neonatal (under 28 days)	44	23	21
Postneonatal (28 days to 1 year)	11	6	5
Infant deaths (under 1 year)	55	29	26

Source: North Carolina Vital Statistics, Division of Health Services, Administrative Services Section, Public Health Statistics Branch, 1976.

COMPARISONS OF FARMVILLE AND
SOUTHERN CITY FAMILY PLANNING PROGRAMS

It is not possible to present more comparable statistics on these
two programs because the Southern City family planning clinic did not
participate in the statewide family planning reporting system, and the
two programs had different data assumptions and analyses. An estimate
of the percentage of women served who were residents of Southern City
is given in Table 6.6. It appears that approximately 12.5 percent of
the estimated number of women ages 15 to 19 in need of family planning
services are being served. In order to obtain some comparative statistics, we calculated the birthrates for all teenage women in Farmville
and Southern City from 1973 through 1976. For 1976 we calculated in
addition the birthrates for teenage residents of Farmville and Southern
City by marital status and race.

From 1973 to 1976 Farmville birthrates exceeded those in Southern City. The percentage increase of Farmville birthrates over those
in Southern City varied from 173 percent in 1975 to 92 percent in 1976.
(See Table 6.7.) Farmville teenagers were having about twice as many
babies per 1,000 females aged 15 to 19 as teenagers in Southern City.
It is not surprising to find that birthrates were higher in the rural and
lower in the urban setting. However, we saw in Chapter 5 that teenagers in both communities wanted only one-fourth of the babies born to
them. Teenagers in Farmville were managing their fertility about half
as successfully as Southern City teens: they were producing twice as
many babies while desiring nearly identical levels of fertility.

There probably is some differential in desired fertility for teenagers raised in Farmville, who may actually want more births. We
know through our survey efforts that teenagers in both communities experienced unwanted fertility at the rate of three unwanted babies for
every one wanted baby born. When calculated in numbers per 1,000 (on
a rate basis), we can say that Farmville's teenage mothers were producing unwanted births at twice the rate of Southern City teenagers.
Table 6.8 shows birthrates for young women aged 13 to 19 in both communities, by race and marital status, for 1976. White teenagers in
Farmville were having legitimate babies at two to three times the rates
of teenagers in Southern City. Black teenagers aged 18 and younger
also were having legitimate births at a rate approximately twice that of
black teenagers in Southern City. White Farmville teenagers in 1976
had out-of-wedlock births at rates only slightly higher than those of
teenagers in Southern City. Those having the most difficult time managing their fertility were black teenagers in Farmville, who in 1976
gave birth at more than twice the rate of black teenagers in Southern
City at ages 14 and 16 and at nearly twice the rate for 15-year-olds.

The Family Planning Evaluation Branch of the Department of
Health, Education and Welfare's Center for Disease Control in Atlanta

TABLE 6.6

Percent of Female Residents Aged 15 to 44 Actively Enrolled in
Public Health Department Family Planning Program, Southern City,
1974

Age	Estimated Number of Women in Need	Number Enrolled, May 1974	Percent Estimated Enrolled
15 to 19	12,232	1,527	12.5
20 to 24	12,339	2,660	21.6
25 to 29	11,170	989	8.9
30 to 34	8,822	342	3.9
35 to 39	7,396	178	2.4
40 to 44	7,084	67	0.9
Total	59,043	5,763	9.8

Source: Southern City Health Department.

TABLE 6.7

Teenage Birthrates, Farmville and Southern City, 1973-76

	Farmville		Southern City		Farmville Birth-rate as Percent Increase over Southern City Birthrate
	Number of Births	Birth-rate	Number of Births	Birth-rate	
1973	167	67	604	28	+139
1974	140	56	577	27	+107
1975	112	45	565	26	+173
1976	121	48	536	25	+92

Note: Birthrate is number of births per 1,000 women in each
age group.

Source: Calculations based on demographic and birth data from
North Carolina Department of Human Resources, Division of Health
Services.

TABLE 6.8

Teenage Birthrates to Residents, by Marital Status and Race, Farmville and Southern City, 1976

Age	Legitimate				Out-of-Wedlock				Farmville Black Out-of-Wedlock Birthrate as Percent Increase or Decrease over Southern City Black Out-of-Wedlock Birthrates
	White		Black		White		Black		
	F	SC	F	SC	F	SC	F	SC	
13						0.5		4	-400
14						0.5	74	21	+252
15	13	3		1		3.0	91	33	+175
16	17	10	12	5	8	5.0	208	54	+285
17	30	18	22	14	4	5.0	143	76	+88
18	64	21	27	15	13	7.0	151	87	+73
19	66	36	12	45	27	25.0	72	66	+10

Note: Birthrate is number of births per 1,000 women in each age group; F = Farmville; SC = Southern City.

Source: Calculations based on demographic and birth data from North Carolina Department of Human Resources, Division of Health Sciences.

estimated that single black teenagers in Farmville were giving birth at a rate 577 percent in excess of their desired rate, while single black teenagers in Southern City were giving birth at a rate 209 percent in excess of their desired rate. White single females in Farmville were estimated by the Center for Disease Control to be giving birth at a rate 600 percent higher than desired; white unwed females in Southern City gave birth at a rate 200 percent in excess of their preferred rate. Thus the actual fertility in both communities was well above the desired levels, with unmarried black teenagers in Farmville experiencing unwanted births 368 percent more often than their Southern City counterparts, and single white Farmville teenagers experiencing unwanted births at a rate 400 percent of that of their counterparts in Southern City. A detailed discussion and an interpretation of these data are given in the section "Value Gaps and Service Gaps" later in this chapter. The point we wish to make here is that numerous teenagers in both communities experienced considerably higher fertility than they desired, according both to the Center for Disease Control and the teenagers themselves.

BARRIERS TO CONTRACEPTIVE USE

Interviews with teenagers suggested a fair amount of ambivalence about sexual activity. Two-thirds of the teen mothers interviewed in both Southern City and Farmville reported that they did not want to become pregnant, yet slightly less than one-third in each group were using any contraceptive methods.

What explanation can be offered for these two apparently contradictory statements? The reasons are many and varied, and the interrelationships are complex. There is the traditional explanation of the hope of preserving a preferred view of oneself as a "good girl" by denying the reality of sexual activity. There is also a prevalent but false belief that a girl cannot get pregnant the first time she has intercourse. Others suggest lack of motivation as well as inadequate knowledge as the basic reasons for poor contraceptive use among adolescents. Since the use of chemical contraceptives has become more widespread, the lack of safety of a particular contraceptive is now more often offered as a reason for not practicing contraception. Yet another reason not often mentioned as a barrier is the accessibility or lack of accessibility to all contraceptive methods.

At the time the field research for this study was conducted in North Carolina, it was illegal for a physician to discuss or dispense contraceptives to anyone under age 18 without written permission of one parent. A year later that law was modified. However, the modification was very limited. It allowed a physician, but only a physician, to discuss and dispense contraceptives to a teenager under 18 without parental permission. The new wording of this law still barred other health and allied health professionals from providing the same information.

Information available to teens in both Farmville and Southern City constituted another stumbling block to getting appropriate contraceptives. Quite regularly we found that the word contraceptive was equated with one specific type of contraceptive, the pill. Only after considerable probing could an interviewer elicit the names and any knowledge of other contraceptive methods. The lack of knowledge about the variety of contraceptive methods, combined with a negative appraisal of the pill, effectively limited options for contraception among teenagers in our study. The girls interviewed generally regarded the pill as unacceptable because of their belief that it caused cancer.

Despite its unpopular representation, the pill is still the most popular contraceptive used by the teenagers studied. Of the 35 teenage mothers interviewed in Southern City, 5 reported they were using the pill. This number constituted almost 50 percent of those using contraceptives in that sample. One difficulty with that figure is that two of the five girls using the pill reported that they used it only sometimes. Without a backup method, using the pill "sometimes" is about as effective as using no contraceptive at all. The sometime use of a contraceptive that must be used regularly is another indication of the teenagers' ambivalence about their behavior.

Side effects of the pill often influence teens to stop taking it. Anita Runyan is a Southern City teenager who had been taking the pill consistently. At one point she began gaining weight. She knew weight gain to be one of the effects some pill takers exhibit and quickly stopped taking the pill, hoping that she would stop gaining weight. Shortly it became evident to her mother and sister that Anita's weight gain was not due to the pill. They knew even before she did that it was a result of an unintended pregnancy. When her mother's and sister's suspicions were confirmed, Anita was very upset. She had tried to act responsibly to avoid becoming pregnant, and she feared that this pregnancy would end her plans to go to college.

What was not clear from the interview with Anita was whether she was one of those few who become pregnant in spite of taking the pill regularly or whether the pregnancy was due to the more probable explanation of human error. Medical researchers today give the contraceptive pill a theoretical effectiveness of 99.6 percent. When the pill is used by all groups of women, the effectiveness drops to 97 percent because of human error such as incorrect counting, forgotten pills, or failure to use a backup method of contraception when pills are forgotten.

In Farmville 6 of the 35 teenage mothers interviewed reported that they were taking the pill as a contraceptive. In this group four girls indicated use of the pill as "sometimes" rather than "always." Again, lack of proper information led to an inappropriate choice. The pill has the drawback of having to be taken every day in order to be effective. For teenagers who are likely to be sexually active only intermittently, it may not be the best method becuase it is hard to sustain the motivation to take a pill each day when, for a period of time ranging from weeks to months, lack of sexual activity may preclude the necessity for taking it. It is also necessary to take the pill for one full cycle (one month) before its effectiveness can be trusted. If sexual activity is intermittent, it is also likely to be spontaneous. Often teenage sexual relationships do not last 28 days, much less allow 28 days for the girl to take the pill as a protective measure.

There was no reported usage of the diaphragm among either Farmville or Southern City teenage mothers. Though the diaphragm is an ancient method of contraception, it is unpopular among teenagers because of the development of chemical and other mechanical contraceptives. It is particularly unpopular among teens because it is an intercourse-related method of contraception.

Only one teenager interviewed in Southern City reported ever having used an IUD. There seems to be a prevalent negative attitude toward wearing one. In some instances girls voiced the fear that the IUD would "rip up" their insides. In other instances discussion of the IUD provoked generalized anxiety. No clear explanation could be offered for that anxiety.

The three methods of contraception mentioned above can be obtained only through a prescription from a licensed physician. While this is not a difficult task, it does entail a visit to a physician, a Health Department, or other health care provider. In making an appointment and following through with the medical visit, a girl faces all the issues of confidentiality, admitting her own sexual behavior, and dealing with an uncomfortable subject with a person who is older, usually a member of the opposite sex, and in a position of superior power (see a discussion of this topic in Chapter 7). Nonprescription contraceptives are easier for teens to obtain for intermittent use. The two primary methods in this category are condoms and spermicidal foams. These may be used alone or in combination with one another. When used in combination, they have a superior effectiveness as a contraceptive.

Despite their good qualities, condoms are used rather infrequently. In Southern City two teenage mothers reported that their partners sometimes used condoms. In Farmville condoms enjoyed even less popularity: no partners had used condoms. One girl each in Southern City and Farmville used foam as a continuous method of birth control. Another teenager in Southern City indicated that she sometimes used foam. However, the foam users and the condom users were not the same persons. While using either contraceptive method is certainly more effective than using none, the effectiveness of either method used alone is considerably less than that of the two used together.

Four girls reported using rhythm as a method of contraception. This method of counting the days of the cycle and abstaining from intercourse during the fertile period can work well for women who have very regular cycles. However, it is not recommended for younger women because their menstrual cycles usually have not achieved that degree of regularity. In addition, the use of rhythm requires strong willpower and a firm commitment to its correct use.

Three of the four girls who reported using rhythm in Farmville and Southern City have reported that they used rhythm only sometimes. One might be tempted to defend their definition of <u>sometimes</u>, except that all of them were selected to participate in the study because they had recently been pregnant. The use of rhythm on a "sometimes" basis suggests two things: either one of the two partners lacked the necessary willpower and commitment or one or both lacked an adequate understanding of the reproductive cycle and the role of contraception in preventing fertilization of an egg.

Sally Martin was one of the teenagers using rhythm because she did not want to become pregnant. The problem with her use of rhythm as a contraceptive method was neatly summarized in her own words: "I always heard about birth control but I didn't know what it was. When they be telling me about birth control, they be telling me about getting checked and hurting. I was scared. I heard too that birth control can make you sick. They say you can still get pregnant if you miss one day." Sally also explained that she did not use the pill because she had never heard of it at the time she got pregnant.

It is clear from these comments that Sally had very limited information with which to make her decisions and on which to pattern her behavior. Largely because of limited availability of information on sex and the reproductive cycle, and the role of contraceptives in preventing pregnancy, Sally was a mother at the age of 14.

The data collected on contraceptives, access to them, and their use in Farmville and Southern City suggest that much more needs to be done in this area in both locales. Not only is there inadequate use of contraceptives; there is also a trememdous gap in the information available to teenagers. Some people question making birth control information available to younger adolescents, but it has not been demonstrated that making the information available will induce them to have intercourse that they would not otherwise have had. Younger adolescents are having intercourse, and without the proper knowledge of human reproduction and birth control. If information regarding the reproductive cycle and the role of contraceptives could be given in a way that met both the emotional and the physical needs of teenagers, there would be hope that they could be more responsible for their sexual behavior.

CONTRACEPTIVES FOR TEENAGERS:
HOW PEOPLE FELT

How do the values held by the groups in our study compare with standards set by the American Public Health Association (APHA)? The APHA calls for giving teens access to contraceptives unrestricted by financial considerations or parental consent. To assess feelings of the two communities, state policy makers, and federal policy makers, we asked three questions that are discussed below:

1. How much do you personally favor or oppose a policy of making contraceptive advice and services available to all teenagers?

2. How much do you personally favor or oppose a policy of providing teenagers contraceptive care without parental consent, if necessary?

3. How much do you personally favor or oppose a policy of providing program funding so that the teenager can easily get contraceptive and abortion services?

Even more dramatically than for the abortion questions discussed in Chapter 5, three distinct groups emerged. Service providers were clearly distinguishable as a group with homogeneous attitudes at all four levels. Policy makers in the two communities (such as board members), in the state government (judges, legislators), and in the federal government (congressmen) formed a second identifiable group distinct from service providers and the third group, the general public. Views of the general public ranged within a narrow enough band to make the public a separate and identifiable group.

As with the abortion data in Chapter 5, the responses of the groups presented in this chapter must be evaluated according to the subjective beliefs of the readers about the meaning of the responses. Our yardstick for evaluating the responses was the standard set in the professional community: full access to contraceptives for all teenagers, regardless of age or ability to pay and without requiring parental consent.

Making Contraceptive Services Available
to All Teenagers

The following are the experiences of one Farmville teenage
mother who tried to get contraceptive services. The circumstances
in which Patti Davis found herself when she became pregnant at 16
were unusual. The very unusualness of her life situation accents the
need for appropriate services to adolescent females. Patti's father
is an alcoholic and her mother has six other children to raise by herself, so Patti was raised in a children's home. Her boyfriend, with
whom she had been "going steady" since she was 11 years old, was
also a resident of the home. Ted is an orphan whose parents had died
in an automobile accident when he was very young. In their will they
had left him a substantial amount of money, which would be his at the
age of 18 if he did not marry before that time. Patti had been having
unprotected intercourse since she was 13 years old. When she discovered she was pregnant at the age of 16, she had no support and no
one to help her deal with her dilemma. In her own words, the best
alternative that she could think of was "going crazy." Ted's advice
was, "Have an abortion—do something to get rid of it." When pushed
to suggest places or persons to whom she could go for help, he suggested finding another man and blaming it on him. Patti's sister's
advice was even more terrifying: drink something to kill the baby.
Patti said that both her sister and her grandmother had done that to
rid themselves of unwanted pregnancies. Her mother suggested that
she go to a home for unwed mothers. However, Patti did not know
where there was one. Her father said that she could stay with him,
but that he had no idea what she should do. The children's home had
no provisions for caring for pregnant women, so Patti had to leave.
    Patti had not been using any contraceptives because her efforts
to get them had failed. She had tried both the Health Department and
social services, and was told by both that she was to young to get
them without her mother's signature.
    Patti is married now to a man four years her senior. Jack has
adopted his wife's daughter and given her his surname. Their chief
worry now is how and when to tell little Jessica the true story of her
parentage.
    Patti's dream is to become a photographer. She would like to
take the two-year course at the technical institute near her home and
then do free-lance work. Because she has been out of school for more
than a year, she could study for and pass the Graduate Equivalent
Test. Otherwise, she would need two more years to complete her
high school education. Jack has completed only ninth grade. Although
they presently live with his parents, Jack and Patti hope soon to be
able to afford to rent a trailer and have a home of their own.

FIGURE 6.3

Percentage of Resistance* to Proposed Contraceptive Policies for Teenagers, Farmville and Southern City, 1976

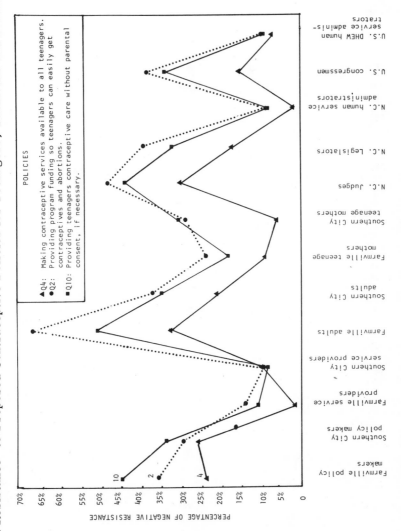

*Resistance is the combined negative response to these three questions.

Source: Constructed by the author.

155

FIGURE 6.4

Attitudes toward a Policy of Making Contraceptive Service Available to All Teens, Farmville, 1977

PERCENTAGE

	Policy Makers (N = 63)	Service Providers (N = 54)	Adult General Public (N = 313)	Teenage Mothers (N = 35)
Favor strongly	0000000000 0000000000 0000000000 0000000	0000000000 0000000000 0000000000 0000000000 0000000000 0000000	0000000000 0000000000 0000000000 0000000	0000000000 0000000000 0000000000 0000000000 0000000000 00
Favor moderately	0000000000 0000000000 00000000	0000000000 0000000000 0000000000 00000000	0000000000 0000000000 00	0000000000 0000000000 0000000
Not sure	0000000000 0	000	00000000	0000000000 00
Oppose moderately	000000000	00	000000000	000000000
Oppose strongly	0000000000 00000		0000000000 0000000000 0000	

Note: Each 0 = 1 percent.

Source: Constructed by the author.

156

FIGURE 6.5

Attitudes toward a Policy of Making Contraceptive Service Available to All Teens, Southern City, 1977

PERCENTAGE

	Policy Makers (N = 62)	Service Providers (N = 55)	Adult General Public (N = 309)	Teenage Mothers (N = 35)
Favor strongly	0000000000 0000000000 0000000000 0000000000 0000000000 00000	0000000000 0000000000 0000000000 0000000000 0000000000 00000000	0000000000 0000000000 0000000000 0000000000 0000000000 000	0000000000 0000000000 0000000000 0000000000 0000000000 0000000000 00000000
Favor moderately	0000000000 0	0000000000 0000000000 0000000000 000	0000000000 0000000000 000	0000000000 0000000000
Not sure	00000000	000	000	000
Oppose moderately	0000000000 000	000	000000000	000
Oppose strongly	0000000000 000	000000	0000000000 00	000000

Note: Each 0 = 1 percent.

Source: Constructed by the author.

FIGURE 6.6

State and Federal Decision Makers' Attitudes toward a Policy of Making Contraceptive Service Available to All Teens, 1977

	North Carolina Judges (N = 125)	North Carolina Legislators (N = 101)	North Carolina HSAs (N = 58)	U.S. Congressmen (N = 83)	HEW* (N = 43)
Favor strongly	0000000000 0000000000 0000000	0000000000 0000000000 0000000000 000000	0000000000 0000000000 0000000000 0000000000 0000000000 000000000	0000000000 0000000000 0000000000 0000000000 00000	0000000000 0000000000 0000000000 0000000000 0000000000 0000000000 0000000000 000000000
Favor moderately	0000000000 0000000000 0000000000 00	0000000000 0000000000 0000000000 00000000	0000000000 0000000000 00000	0000000000 0000000000 00000000	0000000000 0000
Not sure	0000000000 0	0000000000	0000	0000000000 0	
Oppose moderately	0000000000 0000	0000000000	00	0000000000 0	0000000
Oppose strongly	0000000000 000000	0000000		00000	0000000

*HEW = Department of Health, Education and Welfare human services administrators.

Note: Each 0 = 1 percent.

Source: Constructed by the author.

158

If there were health care facilities among whose particular concerns were teenage girls, or if an exception had been made to the law requiring parental consent before dispensing contraceptives to minors, Patti might be a good deal closer to her goal of becoming a photographer.

How do our study communities feel about making contraceptives readily available to teenagers like Patti? A summary overview of the percentage of resistance among all respondents to the three questions concerning the availability and conditions of availability of contraceptives to teenagers appears in Figure 6.3. The full set of responses appears in Figures 6.4-6.6.

In our view, strong support for making contraceptives available to teenagers existed among all groups in both Farmville and Southern City. This level of support continued among state judges, legislators, and human services administrators, and was present among the national congressmen and federal human services administrators in the study (Figure 6.6).

Figure 6.3 shows that on the average, about one-fourth of the policy makers and one-third of the Farmville general public either moderately or strongly opposed a policy of providing teenagers access to contraceptives. Southern City residents showed a varied pattern of slightly more resistance to the idea among policy makers and service providers and measurably less resistance among the general public. Attitudes among the general public were consistently homogeneous with two exceptions: (1) especially strong support for the policy came from Farmville women who had themselves given birth as teenagers and (2) Farmville women who had been pregnant when they married were significantly more supportive of making contraceptives available to teenagers.

Providing Program Funding for Easy
Access to Contraceptives and Abortions

One of our main research objectives was to measure attitudes toward various degrees of birth control availability for teenagers in the two communities. To accomplish this we posed a composite question that went beyond asking the respondent to evaluate a policy allowing contraceptives to be available to teenagers in Farmville and Southern City. The concepts of providing program funding to enable teenagers to get contraceptives "easily" and obtaining abortions easily are added to the question. In sum, this question tested for at least three potentially sensitive policy issues: providing funds for contraceptives for teenagers, making contraceptives "easily available," and providing funding and easy access to abortions for teenagers. We purposely loaded a single question very heavily to measure cumulative resistance.

FIGURE 6.7

Attitudes toward a Policy of Program Funding to Provide Teens Easy Access to Local Contraceptive and Abortion Services, Farmville, 1977

PERCENTAGE

	Policy Makers (N = 63)	Service Providers (N = 54)	Adult General Public (N = 313)	Teenage Mothers (N = 35)
Favor strongly	0000000000 0000000000 00000000	0000000000 0000000000 0000000000 0000000000 00000000	0000000000 00	0000000000 0000000000 0000000000 000
Favor moderately	0000000000 0000000000 000	0000000000 0000000000 0000000000 00000000	0000000000 0	0000000000 00000
Not sure	0000000000 000		0000000000 0	0000000000 0000000000 00000000
Oppose moderately	0000000000 0000000000 000	0000000000 0	0000000000 00000000	0000000000 00
Oppose strongly	0000000000 000	000	0000000000 0000000000 0000000000 00000000	0000000000 00

Note: Each 0 = 1 percent.

Source: Constructed by the author.

160

FIGURE 6.8

Attitudes toward a Policy of Program Funding to Provide Teens Easy Access to Local Contraceptive and Abortion Services, Southern City, 1977

PERCENTAGE

	Policy Makers (N = 62)	Service Providers (N = 55)	Adult General Public (N = 309)	Teenage Mothers (N = 35)
Favor strongly	0000000000 0000000000 0000000000 0000	0000000000 0000000000 0000000000 0000000000 0000000000 000000	0000000000 0000000000 00000	0000000000 0000000000 0000000000 0000000000 0000
Favor moderately	0000000000 00000000	0000000000 000000000	0000000000 0000000000 000000	0000000000 00000
Not sure	0000000000 00000000	0000000000 000000	0000000000 00	0000000000 00
Oppose moderately	0000000000 0	000	0000000000 000	0000000000
Oppose strongly	0000000000 0000000000	000000	0000000000 0000000000 0000	0000000000 0000000000

Note: Each 0 = 1 percent.

Source: Constructed by the author.

FIGURE 6.9

State and Federal Decision Makers' Attitudes toward a Policy of Program Funding to Provide Teens Easy Access to Contraception and Abortion Services, 1977

PERCENTAGE

	North Carolina Judges (N = 125)	North Carolina Legislators (N = 101)	North Carolina HSAs (N = 58)	U.S. Congressmen (N = 83)	HEW* (N = 43)
Favor strongly	0000000000 0000000000 0000000000 000000	0000000000 000000	0000000000 0000000000 0000000000 0000000000 0000000000 000	0000000000 0000000000 0000000000 00000	0000000000 0000000000 0000000000 0000000000 0000000000 0000000000 000
Favor moderately	0000000000 0000000000 0000000000	0000000000 0000000000 0000000000 00	0000000000 0000000000 0	0000000000 0000000000	0000000000 0000000000 00000
Not sure	0000000	0000000000 000	0000000000 00000000	0000000	00
Oppose moderately	0000000000 0000000	0000000000 0000000000 00000000	0000000	0000000000 00000000	0000000
Oppose strongly	0000000000 0000000000 0000000000 0	0000000000 0		0000000000 0000000000	00

*HEW = Department of Health, Education and Welfare human services administrators.

Note: Each 0 = 1 percent.

Source: Constructed by the author.

As might be expected, the level of support for this policy proposal involving public funding, readily available contraceptives, and easy access to abortions was lower than for simply making contraceptives available to teenagers. Even so, as Figures 6.7 and 6.8 show, over half the policy makers in the communities supported the proposal. Support remained strong among service providers, but public resistance rose markedly, especially in Farmville.

Responses of state and federal officials are given in Figure 6.9. Perhaps the best way to depict the increased level of resistance to the policy proposal that provides extensive birth control support for teenagers is to return to Figure 6.4. Resistance rose by 12 percent among Farmville policy makers and by an equal percentage among Farmville service providers. The sharpest rise in resistance was among the Farmville general public, who doubled their resistance level from 33 percent resisting the idea of making contraceptives available to 66 percent resisting the policy of funding both contraceptives and abortions. Resistance among the Southern City public was much more moderate, rising from 21 percent against making contraceptives available to 37 percent opposing a policy of funding contraceptives and abortions.

Cross tabulations of responses of the general public in Farmville reveal that the sources of strongest resistance to the policy of funding contraceptives and abortions were conservative Protestants and persons with high school or less than high school education.

Providing Contraceptive Care to Teenagers
without Parental Consent, If Necessary

Except for policy makers in Farmville and Southern City, most groups of respondents were slightly less resistant to contraceptive care for teenagers without parental consent than to funding contraception and abortions. The detailed responses are given in Figures 6.10-6.12. Responses were surprisingly homogeneous in both Farmville and Southern City. In Farmville there was a tendency for men more often than women to oppose a policy of letting teenagers get contraceptives without parental consent. This finding corresponds to the strong disapproval of early pregnancy expressed by fathers of the teens interviewed. In Southern City resistance was greatest among older respondents in the general public and among women who were not pregnant at the time they were married.

FIGURE 6.10

Attitudes toward a Policy of Allowing Teen Contraceptive Care without Parental Consent, if Necessary, Farmville, 1977

PERCENTAGE

	Policy Makers (N = 63)	Service Providers (N = 54)	Adult General Public (N = 313)	Teenage Mothers (N = 35)
Favor strongly	0000000000 0000000	0000000000 0000000000 0000000000 0000000000 000	0000000000 0000000000	0000000000 0000000000 0000000000 0000000
Favor moderately	0000000000 0000000000 00000000	0000000000 0000000000 0000000000 00000000	0000000000 00000000	0000000000 0000000000 0000000
Not sure	0000000000	00000000	0000000000 0	0000000000 00000000
Oppose moderately	0000000000 000	000000	0000000000 0	000000
Oppose strongly	0000000000 0000000000 0000000000 00	00000	0000000000 0000000000 0000000000 0000000000	0000000000 00000000

Note: Each 0 = 1 percent.

Source: Constructed by the author.

FIGURE 6.11

Attitudes toward a Policy of Allowing Teen Contraceptive Care without Parental Consent, if Necessary, Southern City, 1977

PERCENTAGE

	Policy Makers (N = 62)	Service Providers (N = 55)	Adult General Public (N = 309)	Teenage Mothers (N = 35)
Favor strongly	0000000000 0000000000 000000000	0000000000 0000000000 0000000000 0000000000 0000000000 0000000000 0000	0000000000 0000000000 00000	0000000000 0000000000 0000000000 0000000000 000000
Favor moderately	0000000000 0000000000 0000000000 00	0000000000 00000000	0000000000 0000000000 00000000	0000000000 00000
Not sure	00000	000000000	0000000000 00	000000000
Oppose moderately	0000000000 000	000000000	0000000000 00	000000000
Oppose strongly	0000000000 0000000000 0		0000000000 0000000000 000	0000000000 0000000000 0000000000

Note: Each 0 = 1 percent.

Source: Constructed by the author.

165

FIGURE 6.12

State and Federal Decision Makers' Attitudes toward a Policy of Allowing Teen Contraceptive Care without Parental Consent, if Necessary, 1977

	North Carolina Judges (N = 125)	North Carolina Legislators (N = 101)	North Carolina HSAs (N = 58)	U.S. Congressmen (N = 83)	HEW* (N = 43)
Favor strongly	0000000000 0000000000 0000000000 0000000	0000000000 0000000000 00000	0000000000 0000000000 0000000000 0000000000 0000000000 0000000000 0000000000	0000000000 0000000000 0	0000000000 0000000000 0000000000 0000000000 0000000000 000000000
Favor moderately	0000000000 0000000000 0000000000	0000000000 0000000000 0000000000	0000000000 0000000000	0000000000 0000000000 0000000000 00000000	0000000000 0000000000 0000000000
Not sure	000000000	0000000000 000	00	0000000	00
Oppose moderately	0000000000 000000	0000000000 0000000000 0	00000000	0000000000 0000000000 000000	0000000
Oppose strongly	0000000000 0000000000 00000000	0000000000 0		00000000	00

*HEW = Department of Health, Education and Welfare human services administrators.

Note: Each 0 = 1 percent.

Source: Constructed by the author.

Local, State, and National Comparisons

The homogeneity of attitudes among persons and groups we studied is one of the most interesting sets of results obtained in this study. As mentioned earlier, service providers' attitudes toward these policies were remarkably similar whether the individual was working in Farmville or Southern City, or at the state or federal level. (See Table 6.9.) Service providers showed virtually no resistance to a policy of making contraceptives available to teenagers. Service providers also were comfortable with the policies of providing funds for contraceptives and abortions and of providing contraceptives without parental consent. Nearly 80 percent of the service providers who participated in our study, regardless of level, favored all of these policies.

Local, state, and federal policy makers were consistently less likely than service providers to support full access to birth control services for teenagers. It made more difference to policy makers if the funding of contraceptives and abortions was added to a generalized policy of making contraceptives available to teenagers. Support from policy makers dropped off much more sharply than support from service providers who saw the need for funding.

TABLE 6.9

Ranges of Resistance to Policies Making Birth Control Fully Available to Teenagers, Local, State, and Federal Levels, 1977
(percent)

Range of Resistance To	Policy Makers	Service Providers	Local General Public
Making contraceptives available	16 to 30	2 to 9	21 to 33
Funding contraceptives and abortions	30 to 48	6 to 14	37 to 66
Contraceptives without parental consent	32 to 45	8 to 11	35 to 51

Source: Compiled by the author.

The range of resistance among policy makers was consistent at all three levels: about one-fourth of the policy makers in the study resisted making contraceptives available at all, and about one-fourth resisted funding contraceptives and abortions. Conversely, this meant that three-fourths of local, state, and federal policy makers in the study did support making contraceptives available to teenagers and favored funding contraceptives and abortions and making contraceptives available without parental consent.

The general public resistance in Farmville and Southern City began at a consistently higher level on all these policy issues and ended at a consistently higher level than those of the policy makers and service providers. Generally speaking, about one-fourth of the general public in the two communities resisted a policy of making contraceptives available, and about half resisted funding contraceptives and abortions and providing contraceptives without parental consent.

Returning briefly to Figure 6.12, we find a pattern for judges across the state to be the most consistently resistant to these policy proposals. State and federal legislators' views were within two percentage points of each other on all three policy questions, with local policy makers being slightly more resistant.

Clearly there was low resistance to a policy of making contraceptives available to teenagers. When this policy was spelled out and made more explicit, with provision of funds for contraceptives and abortions and allowing teenagers to obtain birth control without parental consent resistance increased. What does this mean? The resistance will have various meanings, depending on the assumptions readers carry to the data. Value gaps do exist. There is resistance to the APHA standard calling for full access to birth control for teenagers, including funding for contraceptives and abortions and provision of birth control without parental consent. In a pluralistic and democratic society such as ours, does the probability that a majority of service providers, policy makers, and the general public in the urban community (Southern City) favor these policies mean they ought to be implemented there? Or does it mean that because a majority of the general public in the rural community (Farmville) do not favor funding birth control and abortions, those services should not be provided for teenagers in that community?

VALUE GAPS AND SERVICE GAPS

Lack of National Population Policies

The United States has no defined population policy aimed at either increasing or decreasing the population. Over the past several years the objectives of the family planning programs sponsored by federal, state, and local governments, as well as private family planning groups, seem to have centered on preventing unwanted pregnancies. In a democratic society such as ours, no governmental unit has attempted to decide for teenage women which babies are wanted and which are unwanted. The decision of whether or not a pregnancy is wanted is still left up to the individual.

Proportion of Wanted Pregnancies

What proportion of pregnancies among U.S. teenagers have been wanted? Nationwide studies conducted in 1971 and 1972 by researchers at Johns Hopkins University provided information on the number of babies desired by teenagers aged 15 to 19. The Center for Disease Control, using the Johns Hopkins figures, performed what might be called a needs assessment based on pregnancy outcome. That is, they compared the actual number of births occurring to teenagers with the number of births teenagers said they desired, based on national data. The center was able to provide information on the number of babies actually born to teenagers in Farmville and Southern City and to compare this with the number of babies actually desired: the difference between actual and desired fertility. The responsibility of family planning programs such as those of the Health Departments in Farmville and Southern City is to provide the services necessary to enable residents of the community to prevent unwanted pregnancies.

On the basis of national surveys, the desired age-specific fertility rate for white females aged 15 to 19 is 29 per 1,000; that for black females aged 15 to 19 is 43 per 1,000. The desired out-of-wedlock fertility rate (whether the pregnancy was intended or unintended at the time of conception) for white females aged 15 to 19 is 2 per 1,000; that for black females aged 15 to 19 is 22 per 1,000. These are the actual rates at which U.S. teenagers desire births, and they are an appropriate yardstick by which to judge differences between desired and actual fertility in Farmville and Southern City. For various reasons based on medical and social considerations, the Center for Disease Control staff concluded that the desired number of births to females aged 12 to 14 is zero.

Births in Excess of the Desired Number

Across North Carolina white teenagers had 93 percent more births in 1975 than their desired level. In that same year (the latest year for which data are available) black teenagers in North Carolina

TABLE 6.10

Comparative Fertility Analysis, Farmville and Southern City, 1975

Indicator	Number of Births	Population	Birthrate[a]	Numerical Deviation[b] per 1,000	Percent Deviation[c] per 1,000
Farmville					
Females Aged 15 to 19					
Total	125	1,756	71	40	129
White	52	1,345	39	10	34
Other	73	411	178	135	314
Unmarried females Aged 15 to 19					
Total	70	1,449	48	43	860
White	15	1,080	14	12	600
Other	55	369	149	127	577
Southern City					
Females Aged 15 to 19					
Total	540	13,799	39	8	26
White	223	10,132	22	—	—
Other	317	3,667	86	43	100
Unmarried females Aged 15 to 19					
Total	274	11,425	24	19	380
White	49	8,136	6	4	200
Other	225	3,289	68	46	209

[a]Births per 1,000 women of specific group.
[b]These are numerical deviations from the national desired levels as calculated by the Center for Disease Control in Atlanta, Georgia, in 1977.
[c]The percent deviation for each index in which the actual rate is greater than the desired rate. (Only positive percentages are shown.)

Source: Compiled by the author.

TABLE 6.11

Identified Number of Births above Desired Level, Farmville,
Southern City, and North Carolina, 1975

	Farmville	Southern City	North Carolina
Females Aged 15			
White	3	2	136
Other	4	23	374
Total	7	25	510
Females Aged 15 to 19			
White	13	0	5,341
Other	55	158	5,469
Total	68	158	10,810
Marital births of birth order 4 or more			
White	0	0	102
Other	3	0	610
Total	3	0	712
Total identified excess births			
White	16	2	5,579
Other	62	181	6,453
Total	78	183	12,032

Source: Compiled by the author.

had 160 percent more births than their desired level. The data in
Table 6.10 give the results that the Center for Disease Control found
for Farmville and Southern City.

In Farmville white unmarried women aged 15 to 19 had an actual
birthrate 600 percent greater than the desired level; unwed black
teens had an actual birthrate 577 percent greater than desired. The
corresponding teenage rates in Southern City were 200 percent greater
than desired by unmarried whites and 209 percent greater for unmarried blacks. The actual numbers of births above the desired
level in North Carolina, Farmville, and Southern City are given in
Table 6.11. In Farmville, 78 excess births occurred (16 to white
teenagers, 62 to black teenagers) in 1975. In Southern City that same

year, 183 births (2 to white teenagers, 181 to black teenagers) occurred. When all births to females aged 15 to 19 are considered together, the actual rate in Farmville was 129 percent above the desired rate and the actual rate in Southern City was 26 percent above the desired rate. The differences in the success levels at which teenagers were managing their fertility in these two communities appear to be significant.

Teenagers in Need

    Approaching the problem of family planning program effectiveness differently, the Alan Guttmacher Institute conducted a national survey for the federal government focused on women in need of organized family planning programs. The institute's assessment of needs was based on formulas for determining the number of women in need of organized family planning services who are below 150 percent of poverty, who are below 200 percent of poverty, and who are aged 15 to 19. The results, based on this entirely different approach to analyzing

TABLE 6.12

Women in Need, Patients Served in Organized Program, and Women not Served by Organized Program, Farmville and Southern City, 1975

	Below 150 Percent of Poverty		Below 200 Percent of Poverty		Females Aged 15 to 19	
	F	SC	F	SC	F	SC
Women in need	1,407	7,522	2,218	11,442	696	4,352
Patients served	386	5,208	453	6,118	145	3,668
Difference	1,021	2,314	1,765	5,324	551	684
Percent not served	72.6	30.8	79.6	46.5	79.2	15.7

Note: F = Farmville; SC = Southern City.

Source: Compiled by the author.

the family planning program effectiveness in Farmville and Southern City, reconfirm the findings of the Center for Disease Control (see Table 6.12). In 1975, 79.2 percent of Farmville teenagers in need were not served, while the percentage not served in Southern City that year was 15.7.

SUMMARY

Policy makers, service providers, and the general public in both communities knew less about the availability of contraceptive services than about the availability of abortion services. Contraceptive program services in Southern City were readily available to teenagers and did not require parental consent. Contraceptive program services in Farmville were relatively difficult for teenagers to gain access to and required parental consent. Farmville teenagers were having about twice as many babies per 1,000 females aged 15 to 19 as teenagers in Southern City. Yet teenagers in both communities desired nearly identical levels of fertility. Strong support for making contraceptives available to teenagers existed among all groups in both Farmville and Southern City. Providing program funding and not requiring parental consent were less favored than the general policy of making contraceptives available to all teenagers. Unmarried women aged 15 to 19 in Farmville had an actual birthrate nearly 600 percent greater than the desired level, three times higher than the rate among women aged 15 to 19 in Southern City.

In Chapter 9 we will give our interpretation of some of the causes of these radically differing levels of program effectiveness in Farmville and Southern City. Before discussing possible causes for such different levels of effectiveness, two important additional sets of data must be examined: teen access to prenatal care and sex education in Farmville and Southern City.

7

TEEN ACCESS TO PRENATAL CARE

Regular prenatal care is important for a healthy birth to a woman of any age; but because the adolescent body is not yet fully mature, and therefore has growth needs of its own, careful monitoring is even more crucial in teenage pregnancies. For a number of reasons, ranging from denial of the pregnancy to ignorance of health care alternatives to lack of support by family and other community members, teenagers rank higher than average for low prenatal care.

One of the reasons that teenage births are so often classed as high risk is inadequate prenatal care. Medical professionals often comment that the first time a pregnant teenager is seen professionally is when she arrives at the hospital in full labor. In such a situation, any type of patient education is clearly too late. Furthermore, the opportunity has been lost to monitor food intake, to test for vitamin and iron deficiencies, to check blood pressure, and to watch for indicators of toxemia. Nor has the physician had time or opportunity to give a pelvic exam in order to assess size and bone structure.

In both Farmville and Southern City there were teens who received no prenatal care. In Southern City six teenagers received no prenatal care. Another 10 or 11 did not begin prenatal care until the third trimester. Though these numbers seem small, they constitute 12 percent of the cohort of teens who gave birth in Southern City in 1976. Comparable figures are available for Farmville during the same period. There, state records indicate, three girls aged 18 and under—4 percent of the sample—received no prenatal care (see Table 7.1). Six more girls did not begin prenatal care until their third trimester. The total of Farmville girls receiving no prenatal care or beginning their care as late as the third trimester was 12 percent of the cohort.

174

TABLE 7.1

Numbers and Percentages of Teens Receiving No Prenatal Care or
Beginning Care in the Third Trimester of Pregnancy, Farmville
and Southern City, 1976

Prenatal Care Begun	Farmville		Southern City	
	Number	Percent	Number	Percent
Seventh month	0	0	8	5.0
Eighth month	4	5.4	1	1.6
Ninth month	2	2.7	2	1.3
None received	3	4.3	6	3.8
Total in cohort	74		157	

Source: Compiled by the author.

On the other hand, 45 percent of the girls in Southern City and
slightly over 50 percent of the girls in Farmville did seek prenatal
care during their first trimester of pregnancy. One would hope that
each of these girls not only started care early in her pregnancy but
also received consistent and continued care throughout the pregnancy.
However, Health Department records indicate that this was not the
case. For example, in Southern City two girls who started prenatal
care in the first month of their pregnancy had only five visits.

One model of proper prenatal care uses the following pattern of
patient visits. During the first seven months a woman is seen once
a month. During the eighth month she is seen every two weeks. During the last four to six weeks she is seen every week. Depending on
how close to her actual due date the woman delivers, this model suggests 13 to 15 prenatal visits as appropriate for a woman who begins
care in the first month. (To arrive at the appropriate number of
visits for a woman beginning prenatal care later in the first trimester
or the second trimester months, one subtracts the number of months
of pregnancy already completed from the total number of recommended
visits. For example, if a woman began care in the third month of her
pregnancy, then she would subtract 2, making her appropriate number
of visits from 11 to 13.)

On the basis of the model, it is clear that few Southern City
teenagers had consistent prenatal care. Other Southern City exam-
ples confirm the inadequacy of prenatal care. One teen who began

TABLE 7.2

Number of Visits Made by Teens Who Began Prenatal Care in the First Trimester, Farmville and Southern City, 1976

	2	3	4	5	6	7	8	9	10	11	12	13	14	15	16	17 or More	Total
Farmville																	
First month									1		1						2
Second month				2	1		2		3	1	3		2	2			16
Third month	1	2		2		3		1	2	1	4	1	1	1		2	22
Total	1	2	0	4	2	3	2	1	6	2	8	1	3	3	0	2	40
Southern City																	
First month				2			2		2		3					1	10
Second month			1	2	2	1	4	2	2	2	3	2	1	4		3	29
Third month	1		2	1	3	2	4	2	7		4	1		1		3	31
Total	1	0	3	5	5	3	10	4	11	2	10	3	1	5	0	7	72*

*While the correct total is 72, information is missing for two teenagers.

Source: Compiled by the author.

her care in the second month made only four prenatal vistis. Four
others who also began prenatal care in the second month made five
or six visits. Yet another girl who began prenatal care in her third
month made only two prenatal visits. In sum, 72 girls in the Southern
City cohort began their prenatal care in the first trimester of pregnancy. On the surface this figure is satisfactory, since it comprises
45 percent of the 1976 cohort. On closer examination it is evident
that 44 of these 72 girls had fewer than the number of prenatal visits
suggested by the model.

Yet to be mentioned are the remaining 55 percent of Southern
City teens. Forty-four percent did not begin prenatal care until the
second trimester of pregnancy. While many women are just beginning
to "show" at this point, by the fourth month the fetus is fully six inches
long. Although most of the growth in terms of size and weight has yet
to occur, formation of the organs, differentiation of body parts, and
initial development of the nervous system have already taken place.

For the girls who began prenatal care in the second trimester,
care could be given to help maintain the growth of the fetus until term.
But much was left to chance because the influences of diet and possible use of tobacco and alcohol had already had their impact during the
first trimester. The critical phases of embryonic development had
already taken place. In too many cases the teenager had no guidance
during this critical period.

The remaining 11 percent of the total cohort waited until the
third trimester to begin care or received no prenatal care at all.
Records indicate a similar experience for Farmville teens. Thirty-
eight (53 percent) of the cohort began their care in the first trimester
(Table 7.2). Again there was a pattern of inconsistent and inadequate
care. For example, two girls who began their care in the second
month of pregnancy made only five prenatal visits. Another, who
also began her care in the second month, made only six visits. Of
those who began their care in the third month, one girl made only two
visits; two other girls made only three visits; and another six made
seven or fewer visits.

Records for Farmville indicate that approximately 32 percent
of the teenagers who delivered there in 1976 began prenatal care in
the second trimester. This percentage accounted for 25 of 75 girls
aged 18 and under who delivered that year.

FACTORS LEADING TO INCONSISTENT CARE

Several questions need to be asked: When a teenager discovers
an unexpected pregnancy, to whom does she turn for help? Why is
there such a high incidence of teenagers starting prenatal care later

than the first trimester? What factors account for the inconsistency of prenatal care once it has begun? These questions are of primary concern to us. For answers we turned to members of the community in both towns.

Perhaps the group best able to answer these questions is the teenagers themselves. When we interviewed the sample of 35 teenage mothers in each of the two cities, we asked them their opinions. This is what they told us.

Because the majority of teens who engage in sexual relations do not intend or want to get pregnant, they are usually upset or embarrassed when they discover they are. Most pregnant teens never dreamed that they would find themselves pregnant. Often the behavior surrounding the discovery of an unexpected pregnancy is unlike any behavior typical of that individual. The embarrassment or anxiety with which the teenager reacts clouds her ability to think rationally. She is upset, and spends little or no time doing something about her condition. Typically, a girl who had no intention of finding herself pregnant responds by being very secretive. For a long time she tells no one of her situation. Then, when she does tell someone, it will likely be a friend, a sister, or perhaps her boyfriend.

Teens who find themselves pregnant either by choice or by accident have to decide whether to seek professional help. Data indicate that all recorded births in the two study cities occurred in hospitals. Therefore, we know that teens are seeking medical care at some point in their pregnancy. What is unknown is how helpful the persons a teen first tells of her pregnancy are in getting her to seek timely prenatal care. A boyfriend or a girl friend may have no more idea of what should be done than the pregnant teen does. Though these individuals provide needed psychological support, the teenager often is no closer to proper care than before. Because of the high risk associated with early childbearing, this is a cause of concern to medical professionals. However, teenagers seem to be unaware of the importance of prenatal care.

One of the questions asked of teenagers interviewed in this research was, "Who was the first person you told about your pregnancy?" Later the young women were asked who else they told and who they were careful not to tell. Their answers suggested the presence of several patterns that would be of use in the management of adolescent pregnancy in a community. (Though management at this stage is of the pregnancy itself, we assume that similar channels could be used to prevent the occurrence of pregnancy in the first place.)

In general, there were three groups of people to whom pregnant adolescents turned with their problem: boyfriends (or husbands, in the several cases where the teen was married when she became aware of her pregnancy), mothers, and a trusted girl friend. Though boyfriends often were told of the pregnancy before a teen's mother was told, the young woman accepted advice on how to handle her pregnancy more often from her mother than from her boyfriend. Girl friends were in about the same position as boyfriends with respect to offering advice on whom to see for prenatal care or what to do during pregnancy.

Seven teens in Farmville and ten in Southern City listed their fathers as one of the persons whom they told of their pregnancy. However, as reported earlier, the predominant pattern was for a teen's mother to speak to her husband, and then for him and his daughter to have some sort of brief interchange on the subject.

Five of the teens in Farmville talked directly to a family planning worker or a social worker. This number compares unfavorably with the 14 who made the same type of contact in Southern City. One contact was noteworthy in its implied suggestion for outreach workers.

Kate Miller, a rural Farmville teenager, told the interviewer that she had first discussed her probable pregnancy with the public health nurse who came to her home bimonthly to check a sister's high blood pressure. Though this nurse was not identified as a family planning nurse, in this instance she was able to fill that role. Because of her previous contact with the nurse, Kate felt comfortable talking to her and then going to the Farmville Health Department and asking for prenatal care.

It seems important to mention that while all of the teens were attending school at the time their first pregnancy occurred, only one girl in Farmville and four in Southern City chose to talk directly with the school's guidance counselor. Since guidance counselors are on staff at each high school, there seems to be no question of whether they were available or not; rather, it is a question of whether they were perceived as acceptable persons with whom to discuss such a personal issue. As will be mentioned in Chapter 8, sex education conducted in the high schools was usually presented in biology or home economics classes. Therefore, in the teenagers' experiences, the guidance counselor had no prior association with any topic related to sexuality. While these persons are potentially good contact points for referral to health care, the teenagers did not perceive them as such, and so counselors were almost totally neglected.

Unintended Pregnancies

Ronda Smith, a Southern City teenager, was only a little suspicious when her period did not arrive on time. Though she had been having intercourse with her boyfriend and they had not been using a contraceptive, she had been irregular enough in the past that she was not concerned now. It was only after she missed a second period that Ronda became alarmed. At first she did not know what to do. She did what is easiest to do in such a situation: nothing. Finally, when she was about three and a half months pregnant, Ronda told her sister. "Girl, you better go for an abortion. And don't let Mama find out," was her sister's immediate reaction. At the age of 16, Ronda had felt quite mature and wise in the ways of the world. That was three months ago. Now she felt as though her grasp of the world had slipped away from her.

In her fourth month of pregnancy, Ronda finally began prenatal care. Between then and the time she delivered, she made a total of five visits. Her son, born a month early, weighed three pounds, seven ounces.

Francine Jones, a Farmville teenager, was 16 when she became pregnant. She told her boyfriend, Johnny, what she suspected immediately after she missed her first period. His reaction was supportive. "Well, Francine, we can make it. We'll work it out together," he reassured her. He agreed to go with her to tell Mrs. Jones. Francine's mother was disappointed when she heard the news but admitted that everyone "is entitled to one mistake." Because of the large age difference between Francine and her mother, she was inclined to talk more with her boyfriend and a sister who was a year or two older than with her mother.

However, neither Francine nor Johnny had much knowledge of how to handle the pregnancy. Neither knew where to go. Francine's older sister, Tricia, said that she knew some obstetricians in Beaufort, which is nearly an hour's drive from Francine's home. In the end they turned to Mrs. Jones. She had a personal doctor in Farmville. Francine and Johnny went to him, and he recommended an obstetrician.

In this instance the referral to an appropriate person in the medical profession was made by another member of the same profession. Looking back on her pregnancy, Francine was grateful for Johnny's continued support, but she admitted she was not sure she could have done without the help of her family. Even though he wanted to help as much as possible, Johnny was not knowledgeable enough to procure proper care for his girl friend.

An Intended Pregnancy

Other girls reported feeling very proud to discover that they were pregnant. A few of them indicated that they had wanted to get pregnant. Still, wanting to become pregnant does not necessarily imply that a girl has taken any necessary steps toward choosing a physician or obtaining other prenatal care.

Consider the care of Olive Rogers. Olive and her older sister had been adopted by a warm, loving, and religious couple. She had always loved little children, although she had no younger sisters or brothers. As a young teenager she decided she wanted a child of her own. She began to save money and to put away clothes that a baby might use. Before she became pregnant, she had a bank account with enough money to cover what she considered to be the basic costs of an infant. Olive had accumulated this amount over several years. But despite all of this planning for a child, it took Olive three months from the time she first discovered she was pregnant until she began pre-natal care. Despite the certainty with which she went about getting pregnant, she was afraid to tell her mother what she had done. The first doctor she went to thought she was telling a story to gain atten-tion, and refused to give her a pregnancy test. After that refusal it took Olive several weeks to get up her courage to try to convince an-other health care provider that she was pregnant. She finally received a pregnancy test and was told that she was 13 weeks pregnant. Her reaction was, "I could've told them that, if they had just listened."

LACK OF TEEN PARTICIPATION IN THE SYSTEM

The greatest single factor in the delayed start of prenatal care seems to be that teenagers are not participants in the health care sys-tem. Therefore they are not in the habit of making periodic visits to a physician or a clinic. For the most part teenagers we interviewed reported that they knew they could go to the clinic for health care. Some of them also reported that a teenager could go to a private phy-sician. However, very few teens in either Southern City or Farmville had recently visited either of these providers, and therefore felt awkward and unfamiliar when the need to disclose an unplanned preg-nancy arose. In instances where the girl chose to tell her mother early in the pregnancy, and the mother had been making regular visits to either a physician or the clinic, the girl was much more likely to start early prenatal care.

Knowing the facilities exist, knowing how to make an appoint-ment or get medical care, and feeling comfortable in doing so are three very different things. Regardless of when the pregnant teens interviewed started prenatal care, they all knew of at least one place where care could be found. However, knowing that one can get medi-cal care does not mean that a person in need of care will actually seek it. A case in point is a Farmville teenager who had no prenatal care. Joan Grace, age 17, arrived at the emergency room of the hospital late one evening complaining of severe abdominal pains. She was ex-amined and found to be in labor, about to deliver a child. Just past midnight she delivered a five-pound, five-ounce daughter. During labor and delivery, Joan was scared. Because she had had no prenatal care, she had absolutely no idea of what was happening to her body.

Dr. Crane, on call at the Farmville Hospital that night, was scared, too. Because there were no prenatal records, he knew nothing of Joan's physical condition. Since Joan was already well into labor, there was precious little time to make the necessary examinations to determine whether a normal delivery would be possible or safe. Among these tests are evaluation of blood pressure, blood analysis for venereal disease, urinalysis for diabetes or toxemia, and checking the strength of the infant's heartbeat.

Farmville Teenagers

Several girls were so unfamiliar with the appropriate channels for getting good prenatal care that, when asked to list places where they could go for help, the only answer was the Social Services Department. While social services is certainly an entry point to the health care system, lack of knowledge of services provided by the Health Department, hospital, or physicians in Farmville implies an expectation of lack of comfort in dealing with any of these providers for the first time. For the most part girls questioned in Farmville knew of only one place where they could go for prenatal care. If the option was not the Social Services Department or the hospital, then it was either the clinic or a private physician. To many of the girls, both of these last options had more negative than positive features. The clinic had a reputation of asking too many questions and not being very personal. The private doctor had the drawback of being fairly costly for a high school student with no personal income. In several cases the only physician mentioned was the family physician. Going to a person who had been known and used by the family for a number of years caused an added burden to the pregnant teenager, particularly if she had any inclination to have an abortion.

Susan Andrews was another teenager interviewed in our research. She had moved to North Carolina from New York City several years previously. Her family lived in an area where each house was situated on a quarter to half an acre of land. The Andrews family had chosen this part of the county because they had relatives nearby.

When Susan became pregnant, she did not tell anyone at first. In fact, her mother was the first one to suspect. She noticed that Susan had not used any tampons for quite a while. When she approached her daughter and mentioned that fact, Susan smiled shyly and said, "I don't think I'll be needing them for quite some time."

Susan's mother was the one to tell her husband of Susan's pregnancy. While Susan knew that he would not approve of her getting an abortion, there was little other interaction between the two.

Mrs. Andrews had very strong feelings about Susan's prenatal care. She knew of one private physician in the Farmville area to whom she might send her daughter. But her real desire was to have Susan travel to a town an hour from Farmville, where a major medical center was located. Mrs. Andrews's daughter-in-law had had trouble with a pregnancy, and the clinic in Farmville had referred her to that medical center for care. She believed that without adequate care her daughter-in-law might have died. She realized that it was a long way, but she knew that her daughter would receive good care at the center.

Susan also chose to confide in her boyfriend, Sammy, and her sister-in-law, Maggie. Sammy was excited by the pregnancy; he had discouraged Susan from using contraceptives because he wanted her to become pregnant. Now that she was, he suggested that she go to the Farmville clinic for checkups. The clinic was close to his house, and he would be willing to take Susan there for her visits. Maggie also suggested that Susan attend the clinic. She felt that if anything were wrong, the clinic would refer Susan to the medical center. Sammy's willingness to drive Susan to and from appointments, combined with the weight of Maggie's opinion, overcame the strength of Mrs. Andrews's desire to have her daughter receive prenatal care at the medical center an hour away. Susan began prenatal care when she was three months pregnant.

Southern City Teenagers

Teens in Southern City were somewhat more familiar with a range of options for prenatal care. This may be due to the existence of a greater range of options in Southern City than in Farmville or to the teenagers' greater awareness of the options, or both. Most Southern City girls mentioned at least two options, and some as many as three or four. Again, as in Farmville, the clinic and a private physician were the two most frequently mentioned. The difference is that the urban girls often mentioned clinic and physician together. If the girls who had used the health care system were familiar with several options, possibly they were familiar with some of the differences in services offered. If they were unfamiliar with the different services, at least teenagers in Southern City knew who could tell them about health care options.

The lack of knowledge about components of the health care system that could serve the needs of a pregnant adolescent, the attendant lack of comfort in making an appointment to visit any of those places, and the lack of choice for prenatal care services all contribute to the complex issue of why teenagers delay prenatal care until late in their pregnancy.

PROBLEMS IN CONTINUITY OF CARE

Once prenatal care is begun, another set of factors influences the continuity of that care. Some of these problems are specific to the teenager. The most common one is transportation. A number of girls do not have access to cars; others are not yet of legal driving age. One hospital in Southern City recognized this problem and established a program to provide transportation to the prenatal clinic when necessary. Another reason that appointments may be kept irregularly is the teenager's lack of understanding of the importance of good and consistent prenatal care. However, if this awareness does not exist, it seems only logical that the health care provider must impress the reasons for consistent care upon the adolescent.

Girls in both cities were asked to describe the kind of care given to them by the place or person they chose for health care. While some did understand the importance of regular care and were cognizant of the impact of factors such as high blood pressure, diabetes, and sickle cell anemia in their family history, too many girls could only vaguely describe the care given to them. One Farmville teen reported that her family doctor gave her a checkup and provided her with some booklets to read. She also commented that he did not talk to her very much or show any films. The physician most certainly did a thorough physical examination—noting such factors as blood pressure, urine sugar, weight, position and size of fetus, and so forth—and from his point of view the contact was entirely satisfactory. The doctor knew that the pregnancy was progressing normally. However, from the girl's point of view, the contact was unsatisfactory. She had learned nothing from the visit.

Incomplete explanations or no explanations at all are typical of the care that adolescents receive. Explanations are time consuming and often believed to be beyond the teenager's understanding. Therefore, some care providers often give as little explanation as possible. For the teenager there are at least two drawbacks to this type of response: a girl may ask no questions, passively accept the care provided, and learn little or nothing about her pregnancy; without at least some knowledge she can neither care for herself nor report new symptoms to the physician during a routine visit.

A second problem is related to the girl's comfort in seeking and continuing care. If she did not know the physician or people at the

clinic before she came, she knows them no better after her visit.
She feels awkward at having the private parts of her body examined
and at having no idea of what the examination is about. Unless some
of this awkwardness can be eased, there is a higher-than-average
likelihood that the girl will not return on her own initiative.

From another point of view, it might be said that prenatal care
offered in Farmville did not meet the needs of the adolescent seeking
that care. A young teenage mother, Martha Maxwell, had some fairly
strong opinions on the services provided for teens in Farmville:

> The girls here don't know what they're getting into when
> they are pregnant. They go to the doctor and he feels to
> see where the baby is and sometimes checks their blood
> and their urine, but they still have no idea of what they're
> getting into. They need to know something about the birth
> experience itself. They're scared. They've heard stories
> from their mothers and their aunts and other relatives,
> and you know how those stories are. They're really meant
> to scare you, or to tell you how brave that person's been.
> But they still don't know anything even after they've heard
> stories. They need some facts. They need to know what
> they possibly expect. Some of my friends in Southern City
> say that they've seen films—films about childbirth, you
> know, about where the baby comes out and all while you're
> watching the movie. Those are hard for some people to
> watch, but I think it's worthwhile. And they should bring
> the guys, too, for the guys need to know some of the things
> a woman is going through. And he can't appreciate what a
> woman is going through unless he knows.

Another young mother, Candy Kent, said that she wished she
had been told something of what to expect after the birth of the child.
She and her husband worried that they might not be doing the right
thing for their son. Some days she said it seemed impossible to figure out what he wanted. "When he was little, he cried a lot, and I
didn't know what to do for him. It upset me a lot that he was crying,
and probably even more because I couldn't make him stop."

Had Candy and her husband learned something about infant care
before the baby was born, those early months might have been a little
easier for them. They would have known that many babies are colicky
and cry a lot in the first weeks of life. The experience would probably still have been nerve-racking to both of them, but they would
have had a sense of confidence that they had done what they could for
the baby.

In Southern City prenatal care has been adapted to include more
of the needs of adolescents. A number of girls reported seeing films

of the birth experience; some had been involved in prenatal classes where the emphasis was on participation in delivery; and several others reported having seen a film on contraception. Each of these channels of information correctly anticipated at least a part of the adolescent's need. One 17-year-old girl, Mindy East, described in detail the care she received, the films she had seen, and the classes she had attended. She summed up her impression of that care by saying, "They told us what things we needed to know." Though Mindy may not have been able to list those things unless they had been provided for her, it was obvious that the provision of care in this instance did meet the felt needs of the adolescent. This 17-year-old began her prenatal care in the second month of pregnancy and made a total of 15 visits before she delivered a seven-pound, nine-ounce son. Perhaps not all girls would keep all appointments even if their needs were met, but this example does tend to highlight what can happen to the consistency of prenatal care when that care is developed with an understanding of the needs of the adolescent.

8

ACCESS TO SEX EDUCATION

> Sex education comes from peers, other kids or other
> outsiders.
>
> A Farmville physician

Sex education is a difficult concept to define. Understanding
and managing one's sexuality is a lifelong process for most persons.
For the youth in Farmville and Southern City, as in most U.S. communities, the process begins early in life and undergoes a sudden
surge of interest at the onset of adolescence. Our discussion of teenage sexually related needs broadens in this chapter. Abortions, discussed in Chapter 5, are, for most teenagers, one evidence of failure
to manage their fertility according to their own wishes. The effort to
obtain and use contraceptives is a major step that sexually active
adolescents can take toward avoiding abortions and achieving control
over their fertility. In this chapter we examine community and individual efforts to shape an environment in which teenagers can learn
about their sexuality and manage it more successfully.

As was true in the earlier chapters, it has been easier to obtain
detailed information for Farmville than for Southern City, which is
much larger and more diverse. Although there are no data bases for
Southern City comparable in detail with Farmville's, we do have enough
data on Southern City to make meaningful and useful comparisons between the two communities. Not surprisingly, as we have demonstrated in the earlier chapters, the trends in the two communities'
behaviors related to managing adolescent fertility reveal consistent
patterns of involvement in Southern City and noninvolvement in Farmville.

There are a number of dimensions on which sex education could
be defined. At the cognitive level it can be defined as understanding

human sexuality, especially human reproduction. At a more practical
level sex education might be defined as the preparation necessary for
an individual's functional ability to control personal fertility successfully. Behaviorally this control would lead to avoiding unwanted pregnancies. For the purposes of this study, we will use a minimum definition based on sex education activities in Farmville, where a federally funded health educator worked with the Health Department and the
schools. The health educator offered one-hour sessions on menses,
venereal disease, birth control, adolescent development, and human
reproduction. Thus, we define a minimally adequate exposure to sex
education as including at least four one-hour sessions devoted to adolescent development, human reproduction, birth control, and venereal disease. This definition provides a minimum exposure that, in
our view, could be considered sex education. It by no means guaran-
tees an adequate sex education. Sex education is a complicated process with needs for discussions, question-and-answer sessions, and
time to absorb information and return for more information: in short,
a continual process of exploration of the sexual aspects of one's being.
This process cannot be measured in meaningful units of time. A one-
hour exposure to information on adolescent development, human reproduction, birth control, and venereal disease at least opens the possibilities for the initiation of a dialogue between the growing adolescent
and peers, counselors, and family.

SEX EDUCATION IN FARMVILLE

> Sex education can't come from parents—parents of kids
> freeze up—I haven't seen it work for three generations.
>   A Farmville physician

The Home

When and where does sex education take place in Farmville?
The traditional answer has been that sex education occurs in the
family setting. The evidence we presented in Chapters 3 and 4 leads
us to believe that little, if any, sex education is provided in a majority
of the homes in Farmville. Unquestionably some "sex education" in-
evitably happens in the family setting. However, the adults and the
teenagers in this study both agreed that adolescents and their parents
are not in sufficient communication with each other on the subject of
sex for there to be an adequate level of management of teenage fertility in Farmville. It seems to us reasonable to assert that the
amount of useful sex education that occurs in Farmville homes is
negligible.

The Physicians

If sex education is too awkward to be undertaken successfully in the home, the family physician is commonly thought of as a person who is both equipped to provide sex education and able to do so. It is true that most family physicians are able to offer sex information to young people, and their emotional detachment makes them valuable sources of sex education. One of the surprising facts already reported by us, however, is that the physicians participating in our study did not have time to provide sex education to youths who came to them for birth control help or who simply desired information.

The Churches

Beyond possible help from family and the family physician, the churches are commonly thought of as a good source of advice to teen-agers trying to make successful adjustments to adolescence. While we did not systematically poll each church on its teaching program in the area of sex education, we found no literature in any church's junior high or high school curriculum that approached offering functionally useful information in areas such as adolescent development, human reproduction, birth control, and venereal disease. The literature we were able to review generally discussed sex in terms of temptations to be overcome by channeling sexual energy into sports or other accepted social outlets. The general themes seemed to be along the line that sexual activity before marriage is sinful, so the best way to handle sexual urges is to sublimate them. While there may be some exceptions, the churches are not a major source of sex education.

The Schools

> The community doesn't want sex education in the school
> because they don't want to deal with it and they don't
> trust the school to deal with it properly.
> > A Farmville school official

If sex education does not come from the family because it is too awkward for most parents to deal with, if the doctors are too busy, and if the churches ask the teenagers to sublimate their sexual drives, then the public schools are left as the major community resource for providing a minimum sex education for the youth. The schools have assumed that task with varying degrees of commitment and success.

All categories of people interviewed reported that sex was discussed in biology classes and in some home economics classes. However, what is not clear is the manner in which the topic was discussed. Various methods of discussing sex and the gaps inherent in them will be discussed later in this chapter.

The Farmville school official quoted above believed that parents in the community did not want to deal with their children's sexuality, but neither did they want the schools to teach their children basic values and attitudes toward sex. Below we will discuss whether this official was right. To the extent that he was right, youth in Farmville had only their peers from whom to obtain their sex education.

The High School

> It was not a planned thing [sex education in the Farmville school classroom], it was the abhorrence of one of the teachers of the number of big bellies in her classroom.
>
> A Farmville physician

One distressed classroom teacher in the Farmville high school decided to invite a local physician to lecture on sex and birth control to her students. The physician related that in that year (1974) and in the following year, about 150 to 200 students were brought together for a two- to three-hour session. He stated that some of the students "would not care if a naked female walked through the room, while others were about to do it in the room." The teenage girls in the audience, he observed, ran the gamut "from preachers' daughters who will be frigid to colored girls with two kids already." One thing he learned was "to talk to males and females separately." The teacher did not invite the physician back in 1976. The only high school students to receive sex education in the Farmville high school in 1976 were 8 trainable and 15 educable mentally retarded students.

A common assumption is that sex education occurs in the health, home economics, and biology classes of the schools. However, when we interviewed the school counselors and principals, we learned that occasionally a home economics teacher in one or two of the schools will talk about sex in her classes, and that occasionally a science teacher will mention it in the classroom. Usually these classes are electives; and the amount of information given, while far better than nothing, does not begin to approach coverage of the topics we mentioned as a minimum exposure: human reproduction, adolescent development, birth control, and venereal disease.

When sex is mentioned, it is often too little, too late. One high school counselor said that a biology teacher told her that a student came up after one class session in which human reproduction had been

TABLE 8.1

Estimated Number of Teenagers in Grades 7-12, Farmville, 1976

Grade	Average Age	Number	Less .05*
7	13	686	652
8	14	642	610
9	15	618	587
Total			1,849
10	16	620	589
11	17	610	580
12	18	607	577
Total			1,746
Grand total			3,595

*Allows for dropouts, private school attendees, and other unknown factors possibly reducing the actual number of children attending Farmville schools in 1976.

Source: Compiled by the author.

discussed and said she was glad to learn more about the baby she had a year earlier. When the high school counselors were asked if there was a sex education program in the school, one replied, "I'm sure there must be. A science teacher mentioned it in his class." That a science teacher or a home economics teacher mentions sex in the classroom seems to be a random occurrence in the school system and is common knowledge among the teachers because of its rarity.

The federal government provides a health educator's services to Farmville and a nearby county. The health educator works half time in Farmville, primarily at the Health Department, where she provides individual counseling to women attending the family planning clinic. She contacts all principals and teachers in the Farmville school system each year, offering to come to their classes to provide sex education sessions, as many or as few as the teacher may wish.

The health educator offers one-hour sessions on such subjects as adolescent development, abortion, birth control, menstruation,

TABLE 8.2

Number and Percent of Students in One-Hour Sessions, by Sex Education Topic and Grade, Farmville, 1976

Topic	Grade													
	6		7		8		9		10*		11*		12*	
	Num-ber	Per-cent	Num-ber	Per-cent	Num-ber	Per-cent	Num-ber	Per-cent	Num-ber	Per-cent	Num-ber	Per-cent	Num-ber	Per-cent
Menses	36	11												
Adolescent development														
Male			113	16	122	20	37	6						
Female			105		111	18								
Birth control							125	21						
Human reproduction					51	8								
Venereal disease			63	10	53	9	89	15						
Abortion							15	3						
Percent contacted						4						1.3		

*All mentally retarded students (23 in all) in the high school received one-hour sessions on adolescent development (male and female), birth control, human reproduction, and venereal disease.

Source: Compiled by the author.

venereal disease, and pregnancy and prenatal care. During the school year 1976/77 there were approximately 1,849 students in the seventh, eighth, and ninth grades, and approximately 1,746 students in grades 10, 11, and 12 in Farmville. (See Table 8.1.) Table 8.2 shows the sessions taught, by course and by grade, in Farmville schools in 1976. Remarkably, except for the 8 trainable and the 15 educable mentally retarded high school students, no high school students received any sex education in 1976. The 23 mentally retarded students constituted 1.3 percent of the high school students in the Farmville system that year.

Grades 7-9

When the sex education sessions recorded in Table 8.2 are broken down to individual schools and classes (see Table 8.3), it becomes clear that only three of the nine schools in the system had any organized sex education. Students in two French River ninth grade classes apparently received instruction in adolescent development, venereal disease, and birth control in 1976. There appear to have been 74 students in these classes, which yields a 4 percent sex education rate in the junior high grades in Farmville during 1976. Some of the students at Farmville's York School and Brownsville Middle School received instruction in adolescent development, venereal disease, menstruation, and human reproduction. None of them received any information on birth control. It seems reasonably certain that throughout the Farmville school system in 1976, only the two classes of ninth grade students in French River School received instruction that might meet any minimum definition of sex education. In sum, none of the high school students and only two ninth grade classes in one of Farmville's nine schools received birth control information the year of our study.

The teenagers' reports reaffirmed the above. However, their youth and their lack of experience often clouded the issues for them. Many of them were confused as to whether they had had a course in sex education. This confusion was shown mainly in the case of high school biology. One of the units of the course was undoubtedly reproduction. This unit explained the different organs involved in reproduction and the process by which reproduction takes place. The explanation was clear, yet there seemed to be something missing. One teenager who had thought about the course a great deal put it more clearly than the others could. "They tell you about all the parts and everything, but they don't tell you about the emotions, about the things that people feel." Her comment was echoed time and again. Facts can be clearly and intellectually presented to the youngsters. But within the framework of the biology course, human reproduction

TABLE 8.3

Number of Students in One-Hour Sessions, by Sex Education Topic
and School, Farmville, 1976

Topic	York School	French River School	Brownsville Middle School
Menses	66	96	
Adolescent development			
Male	37		200
Female	26	37	189
Birth control		110	
Human reproduction			51
Venereal disease	63	74	
Abortion			
Percent contacted (for all nine schools)		4	

Note: Only these three schools had any sex education classes.

Source: Compiled by the author.

was something done by a set of organs, not by two people. Relationship was the concept that was never dealt with. How much a girl
should give, when she should stop, and how far to go were questions
on each girl's mind that were never dealt with in biology; and since
policy makers and educators alike saw biology as the only arena, these
issues were never covered.

Peers

The Farmville physician quoted at the beginning of this chapter
is correct. The only significant source of sex education in Farmville
is "other kids."

Beverly Coors and her girl friend regularly discussed what they
called the facts of life. They shared with each other how they thought

people made love and who among their friends they thought had done it. If Beverly's own naiveté in the interview is any indication of the level of knowledge among the girls of her group, one could be certain that discussions never got far beyond vague general statements. Beverly had not learned much about sex at home. She had made several attempts to talk to her mother about sex; her mother always said, "You'll learn." Eventually she did learn—the hard way. She gave birth to a healthy son at the age of 17.

Parents appear to be uncomfortable with the subject of sex, the physicians are too busy to provide information, and the schools are not choosing to provide it. The systematic attempt at sex education for Farmville teenagers did not extend past two ninth grade classes and the mentally retarded students at the high school. One of the high school counselors described it this way: "Everybody is on their own. We're just like a big-time college (here in the high school). If you want it, you ask for it, and if not, you don't get it."

When discussing the availability of birth control services, one social worker commented that the daughters of Aid to Families with Dependent Children (AFDC) mothers received the best help in the county. In terms of being provided a minimum sex education, the advantage went to the trainable or educable mentally retarded pupils in Farmville.

Martha Maxwell, a teenager, had relevant experiences and ideas for sex education programs. She had particularly strong ideas about what types of programs should be provided for adolescents in Farmville and in other areas of North Carolina. She felt strongly that the schools should be used, that they are the best place to give both sex information and counseling to students. She knew a number of girls who needed a place to discuss teenage relationships, the do's and don'ts, contraceptive use, pregnancy, and the like. Martha was realistic in her acceptance that the major burden for contraceptive use still falls on the woman.

Martha was quite emphatic, however, that the young men should be required to attend sex education classes. These classes, she thought, should be separate from those held for the girls. Martha was not sure exactly how well the young men would listen, but she knew that "some would think about it later."

Martha learned a lot through her own early experience with pregnancy. She reported that she had been taking the pill regularly when, at 16, she found herself pregnant. She told her boyfriend Reginald the unexpected news, and together they agreed Martha should have the baby. She still remembers how upset she was when she first realized that she was pregnant. Martha recalled that she felt she had no one to trust, and for quite some time she attempted to keep the pregnancy from everyone except Reginald. In the second month of her pregnancy, Martha had a pregnancy test at the public health clinic. She began prenatal care in the third month and had a total of 11 prenatal visits. She gave birth to a healthy boy in September 1976.

Her second son was born 11 months after the first. She and Reginald have worked out an arrangement whereby he works days while she takes care of the children, and Martha works nights while he cares for them. Despite the burden of having two children while so very young, Martha seems well in control of her situation and is able to listen to and help other girls in the same situation make personally appropriate decisions.

Perhaps because of her own experiences, but also because of her natural empathy, Martha is often called upon to give advice or to help neighborhood teenagers cope with pregnancy. Both black and white girls seek her out to ask advice on what to do about pregnancy, relationships with their boyfriends, how to tell their parents they are pregnant, and what to do after the baby is born.

Martha is well aware of the power of her advice-giving role and is always careful to distinguish between her own position on an issue and the possible alternatives open for others to follow.

One particular instance was particularly difficult for Martha. A young girl, Saundra, who had recently become pregnant came to her. The girl seemed to want to terminate her pregnancy, but was looking for someone to tell her that abortion was the right solution. Martha spent the afternoon with Saundra, sharing the different ways that she might handle her pregnancy. Martha realized that she could not make Saundra's decision for her, nor could she tell her what to do. Saundra had to reach a decision herself. Martha's own position is that she does not believe in abortion, although she can accept the fact that a person might make one mistake and need to have an abortion. However, Martha added, she finds no excuse for having more than one.

Although Martha has completed only nine years of schooling, she plans to continue her role as lay facilitator. "These girls who get pregnant, they have no one to talk to, nowhere to go," she explained. In the course of two pregnancies, Martha found no person and no place in the Farmville area where teens can go to discuss their concern and find a sympathic person who will share both time and information.

SEX EDUCATION IN SOUTHERN CITY

Our impression is that sex education is still difficult for teenagers living in Southern City to find. Our sample of the general public and teenagers indicates the same difficulties as those of Farmville teenagers in obtaining information from parents. Similarly, physicians in Southern City who participated in the study consistently said they referred teenagers to the Health Department clinic and gave little or no sex education themselves.

The Health Department

Public agencies in Southern City, however, have taken steps not yet taken by public agencies in Farmville. For example, when teenagers arrive at the Health Department either to obtain a pregnancy test or to get birth control pills, they receive a pamphlet explaining all the methods and sources of birth control and abortion help. There are three full-time nurses available to talk with the teenagers, as well as audiovisual materials, all funded by the county commissioners. We have no information on sex education efforts by Southern City churches. The denomination materials we reviewed in Farmville are the same types provided to the churches in Southern City.

The School System

For a number of reasons, the detailed data we were able to obtain from Farmville are not available for Southern City. This is so partly because the situation is complex. The Southern City school system began to take active steps toward providing sex education in 1973. In 1974 the school board approved a sex education guide written by a committee of Southern City teachers that included, in addition to sex education, chapters on nutrition, emotional development, first aid, and dental and community health. The sex education chapter called for three weeks of daily class sessions, and begins with fifth graders. Letters were sent to parents telling them about the series and indicating that alternative time uses were available to children whose parents did not wish to have them participate. Four workshops a year were held to familiarize the teachers with the guide and the material on sex education. All teachers were given copies of the guide. In addition, posters were placed in Southern City schools telling teenagers how to seek birth control help from the Health Department.

How many teachers were using the guide, including the sex education materials? The closest we were able to get to an accurate estimate was that of 40 percent made by the health educator responsible for sex education at the Health Department. She also offered lectures in individual Southern City classrooms on the same basis and the same subjects as the health educator in Farmville.

At one elementary school only one teacher used the guide chapter on sex education. She gave reasons why more teachers did not use the materials: (1) the school system did not require a specific amount of time for sex education, so the subject often got squeezed out; (2) the guide was new, and teachers were still unfamiliar with it; (3) teachers who did not feel comfortable with sex education were not expected to tackle it; and (4) some teachers feared adverse public reaction.

Teens interviewed in Southern City had no difficulties stating their views on sex education. They reported a distinct lack of facilities and persons to whom they could go to discuss sex. Time and time again teenagers indicated that they wished there was a service to counsel and teach them about birth control.

Neither Belinda nor Elaine knew about contraceptives in time to prevent her pregnancy. The first indication Belinda had that her body was changing was a feeling of nausea in the early morning. For a long time she believed it was a virus and thought of no other possibilities. Her boyfriend was the first to suspect pregnancy. She did not have a pregnancy test until she was two and a half months pregnant. When pregnancy was confirmed, Belinda and her boyfriend decided to get married so that they would be better able to care for the child. Her mother had wanted her to have an abortion because she did not think Belinda was old enough to accept the responsibility of a baby. Now the child is staying at a day-care nursery close to Belinda's home while the young mother tries to finish high school, but Belinda reports that she finds it very difficult to keep her mind on the subject matter. Every time her little one smiles at her, Belinda is glad she did not have an abortion. Still, she wishes she had known about contraceptives, for she finds it difficult to be a student, a wife, and a mother and succeed in all three roles. Belinda was 15 years old when her baby was born.

Elaine began her pregnancy by sleeping all the time. A friend of her sister's suggested that pregnancy might be the cause of the continual drowsiness. Elaine never suspected pregnancy. She felt that sex education should be offered by the school in classes that are taken by all the students. "People should sit down and talk to you about what's what," said a determined Elaine. For best results she felt sex education should begin early, possibly around the sixth grade.

Another girl, Nalda Martin, had her first baby at age 18. Some of her friends said that they wanted to get pregnant so they could catch a man. Nalda felt strongly that "somebody needs to sit down and talk to these girls." She believed her friends needed to know more about their futures and exactly what they were getting into. She said, "They probably won't want their husbands in five years or so." Nalda thought that young girls should be provided with counseling on contraception and information on childbirth and child rearing. She believed that if girls knew that the road ahead was often hard, they would change their minds about having children so young. "And besides that, having a baby doesn't really catch a man. They only stay around for a few months when the baby is tiny. Then they go on their own way." At that point teenagers are left alone physically, emotionally, and often financially, to raise the infant by themselves.

Other girls felt that in addition to sex education, they needed help with making birth control decisions. These girls were discovering that there was no perfect method of contraception. They needed to know the benefits and risks of each method. There was a general feeling among teens interviewed that birth control should be more easily available to young people. If information and contraceptives were more readily available, the girls thought that more teens would learn about birth control and probably would use contraception. Thus, at least some of the unwanted, unplanned pregnancies could be prevented.

SEX EDUCATION IN FARMVILLE AND SOUTHERN CITY

Farmville

The differences in Farmville's approach and Southern City's approach are significant. According to one long-term member of the Farmville Board of Education, the policy makers and most service providers in Farmville decided to ignore the need for sex education. We agree. Nothing was done by private citizens groups, the boards, or the agencies to begin providing sex education for Farmville teenagers.

Southern City

Southern City, in contrast, began to provide sex education at several levels:

1. The Health Department produced its own pamphlet on birth control methods and abortion. It hired a full-time health educator, paid with county funds, to provide assistance to the Health Department, organizations, and the school system in developing a curriculum in sex education.

2. Posters in the public schools told adolescents where and how to get help.

3. The board of education recognized the need for sex education, and a committee of teachers wrote a guide approved by the school board and distributed to all the teachers.

4. To enable teachers to begin providing sex education in their classrooms, workshops were provided four times a year to help them develop their skills and get over feelings of awkwardness in teaching sex education.

5. The school board, in effect, told teachers who felt unready or were unwilling to teach sex education as part of their classroom work, that they should invite specialists into their classrooms to teach sex education.

Southern City, by its actions, formulated policies and took steps toward recognizing that community management of adolescent pregnancies is a problem that can and should be approached through actions taken by the public and private agencies in the community. The practical results are that in Southern City the Health Department and the school board formulated policy and sought county budget support for sex education and birth control efforts for the community.

Most important, Southern City health officials and school personnel wrote their own guidebooks that, it appears, successfully met community needs in ways sensitive to community mores; hence, opposition was minimal. For example, no parents requested that their children not receive the sex education course offered in the elementary school. In Chapter 9 we will explore some of the administrative impacts of the differing situations in Farmville and Southern City.

SHOULD PUBLIC SCHOOLS PROVIDE TEENAGERS SEX EDUCATION AND FAMILY LIFE EDUCATION?

In both Farmville and Southern City the policy makers, service providers, general public, and teenagers said yes overwhelmingly to providing teenagers with family life and sex education. So did state judges, legislators, human services administrators, congressmen, and Department of Health, Education and Welfare administrators. Figures 8.1-8.3 display the percentages of responses to this question. The only group showing any indecision was the teenage mothers (12 percent undecided). We interpret the virtual absence of opposition from policy makers and service providers in both communities to be decisive. In Farmville only 10 percent of the adult general public responded negatively; in Southern City the rate was 5 percent.

A detailed analysis of the results confirms the clear patterns of responses that have been described in the earlier chapters. Compared with Southern City respondents, about 10 percent fewer Farm-

FIGURE 8.1

Attitudes toward a Policy of Providing Sex Education and Family Life Education in the Local Public Schools, Farmville, 1977

	Policy Makers (N = 63)	Service Providers (N = 54)	Adult General Public (N = 313)	Teenage Mothers (N = 35)
Favor strongly	0000000000 0000000000 0000000000 0000000000 0000000000 0000000000 0000000000 0000000	0000000000 0000000000 0000000000 0000000000 0000000000 0000000000 0000000000 00000000	0000000000 0000000000 0000000000 0000000000 0000000000 0000000000 0000000	0000000000 0000000000 0000000000 0000000000 0000000000 00
Favor moderately	0000000000 0000000	0000000000 000000000	0000000000 000000	0000000000 0000000000 0000000000 0000000
Not sure	0000		00000000	0000000000 00
Oppose moderately			000	
Oppose strongly			0000000	

Note: Each 0 = 1 percent.

Source: Constructed by the author.

201

FIGURE 8.2

Attitudes toward a Policy of Providing Sex Education and Family Life Education in the Local Public Schools, Southern City, 1977

PERCENTAGE

	Policy Makers (N = 62)	Service Providers (N = 55)	Adult General Public (N = 309)	Teenage Mothers (N = 35)
Favor strongly	0000000000 0000000000 0000000000 0000000000 0000000000 0000000000 0000000000 0000000	0000000000 0000000000 0000000000 0000000000 0000000000 0000000000 0000000000 0000000000 0	0000000000 0000000000 0000000000 0000000000 0000000000 0000000000 00000	0000000000 0000000000 0000000000 0000000000 0000000000 0000000000 0000000000
Favor moderately	0000000000	000000000	0000000000 0000000	0000000000 00
Not sure	000		000	0000000000 00
Oppose moderately			00	000
Oppose strongly			000	000

Note: Each 0 = 1 percent.

Source: Constructed by the author.

202

FIGURE 8.3

State and Federal Decision Makers' Attitudes toward a Policy of Providing Sex Education and Family Life Education in the Public Schools, 1977

PERCENTAGE

	North Carolina Judges (N = 125)	North Carolina Legislators (N = 101)	North Carolina HSAs (N = 58)	U.S. Congress-men (N = 83)	HEW* (N = 43)
Favor strongly	0000000000 0000000000 0000000000 0000000000 0000000000 000000	0000000000 0000000000 0000000000 0000000000 0000000000 0000000000	0000000000 0000000000 0000000000 0000000000 0000000000 0000000000 0000000000 0000000000	0000000000 0000000000 0000000000 0000000000 0000000000 000	0000000000 0000000000 0000000000 0000000000 0000000000 0000000000 0000000000 0000000000 0000000000
Favor moderately	0000000000 0000000000 00000	0000000000 0000000000 000	000000	0000000000 0000000000 0000000000 0	0000000000
Not sure	00000	0000	0000	000000	
Oppose moderately	000	00			
Oppose strongly	0	0			

*HEW = Department of Health, Education and Welfare human services administrators.

Note: Each 0 = 1 percent.

Source: Constructed by the author.

ville respondents strongly favored the idea. Human services providers at the local, state, and national levels continued to be the most supportive and to register the least resistance to the idea.

It seems clear to us that there is agreement among the respondent policy makers, service providers, and the general public in the two communities, the state of North Carolina, and on the national level that sex education and family life education are appropriate and desirable additions to the school curriculum. The near unanimity of this feeling is a consistent and logical position, given the widespread recognition among participants that a minimum sex education is not being provided in the family setting and that no other public or private agency or group has filled, or is perceived as likely to fill, the gap. The school systems, on the other hand, seem not to have sensed this.

In structuring the question, Should the schools teach all junior high school students about birth control?, we purposely moved to a fairly extreme circumstance. First, the question deals with birth control, not the more abstract ideas of sexuality or the facts of biology. Second, the question asks if actual courses are acceptable, which conveys the idea of more than brief mention focusing specifically on the topic of preventing births. Third, we asked about the junior high level. Fourth, we introduced the concept of teaching all students.

Although resistance increased among every group of participants except the Southern City teenagers, who showed no resistance to the idea, the increases were, in our judgment, modest (see Figures 8.4 and 8.5). The familiar pattern remains: policy makers and the general public in Farmville were more opposed than their Southern City counterparts. One-fourth of the Farmville policy makers and adult general public resisted this policy. The only group in which more than 10 percent of the study participants were strongly opposed was the Farmville general public. The largest portion of the resistance among the Farmville general public came from the conservative Protestants (48 percent opposed) and the Roman Catholics (43 percent opposed) (see Figure 8.6).

Readers will place different interpretations on the meanings of these results for policy makers, especially for the county commissioners and the school board members. Does the response by 25 percent of the Farmville policy makers and adult general public mean that such a policy should not be considered because it conflicts with a portion of the public's values? In a democracy this is a difficult question to settle. The opposite interpretation of this datum is that 75 percent of all policy makers and the general public, and 90 percent of the service providers and teenagers, favored a policy of teaching birth control to all students in junior high school. State and national support for this policy position was high among all groups,

FIGURE 8.4

Attitudes toward a Policy of Teaching about Birth Control in All Local Junior High Schools, Farmville, 1977

PERCENTAGE

	Policy Makers (N = 63)	Service Providers (N = 54)	Adult General Public (N = 313)	Teenage Mothers (N = 35)
Favor strongly	0000000000 0000000000 0000000000 0000	0000000000 0000000000 0000000000 0000000000 000000000	0000000000 0000000000 0000000000 0000000000 0	0000000000 0000000000 0000000000 0000000000 000
Favor moderately	0000000000 0000000000 00000000	0000000000 0000000000 0000000000 00	0000000000 0000000000	0000000000 0000000
Not sure	0000000000 000	0000000000 0	0000000000 000	0000000000 0000000000 0
Oppose moderately	0000000000 000000000	00000	000000000	0000000000 00
Oppose strongly	000000	000	0000000000 0000000	000000

Note: Each 0 = 1 percent.

Source: Constructed by the author.

FIGURE 8.5

Attitudes toward a Policy of Teaching about Birth Control in All Local Junior High Schools, Southern Ctiy, 1977

PERCENTAGE

	Policy Makers (N = 62)	Service Providers (N = 55)	Adult General Public (N = 309)	Teenage Mothers (N = 35)
Favor strongly	0000000000 0000000000 0000000000 0000000	0000000000 0000000000 0000000000 0000000000 000000	0000000000 0000000000 0000000000 0000000000 00000000	0000000000 0000000000 0000000000 0000000000 0000000000 0000000000 00
Favor moderately	0000000000 0000000000 0000000000 0000000000 00	0000000000 0000000000 0000000000 0000000000 00	0000000000 0000000000 0000	0000000000 0000000
Not sure	00000000	000	000000000	0000000000 00
Oppose moderately	0000000000	0000000000	0000000000 00	
Oppose strongly	000		000000	000000000

Note: Each 0 = 1 percent.

Source: Constructed by the author.

206

FIGURE 8.6

Attitudes of Farmville General Public toward a County Policy of Encouraging Courses about Birth Control for All Students in Junior High School, by Religion, 1977

	Conserva-tive Prot-estant	Mainline Protestant	Roman Catholic	Other
Favor strongly	0000000000 0000000000 0000000000	0000000000 0000000000 0000000000 0000000000 000	0000000000 0000000000 0000000000 0000000000 0000000000 0000000	0000000000 0000000000 0000000000 0000000000
Favor moderately	0000000000 00000	0000000000 0000000000 000		0000000000 0000000000
Not sure	0000000	0000000000 00		0000000000 0000000000
Oppose moderately	0000	0000000000 0		000000000
Oppose strongly	0000000000 0000000000 0000000000 0000000000 0000	0000000000 0	0000000000 0000000000 0000000000 0000000000 000	0000000000 0

PERCENTAGE

Note: Each 0 = 1 percent.

Source: Constructed by the author.

FIGURE 8.7

State and Federal Decision Makers' Attitudes toward a Policy of Teaching about Birth Control in All Junior High Schools, 1977

PERCENTAGE

	North Carolina Judges (N = 125)	North Carolina Legislators (N = 101)	North Carolina HSAs (N = 58)	U.S. Congressmen (N = 83)	HEW* (N = 43)
Favor strongly	0000000000 0000000000 0000000000 000	0000000000 0000000000 0000000000 0000000	0000000000 0000000000 0000000000 0000000000 0000000000 0000000000	0000000000 0000000000 0000000000	0000000000 0000000000 0000000000 0000000000 0000000000 0000000
Favor moderately	0000000000 0000000000 0000000000 00000	0000000000 0000000000 0000000000 000000000	0000000000 00000000	0000000000 0000000000 0000000000 0000	0000000000 0000000000 0000000000 0
Not sure	0000000000	0000000000 00	000000	0000000000 0000000000 0	0000000
Oppose moderately	0000000000 000	00000	000000	0000000000 0	00000
Oppose strongly	000000000	0000000		0000	

*HEW = Department of Health, Education and Welfare human services administrators.

Note: Each 0 = 1 percent.

Source: Constructed by the author.

with the state judges showing the most resistance. Service providers at all three levels gave strong support. (See Figure 8.7.)

VALUE GAPS AND SERVICE GAPS

In 1977 sex education efforts in Farmville reached less than 5 percent of the students. In Southern City between 20 and 40 percent of the students may have been reached. Farmville policy makers and service providers were ignoring the need for sex education in the schools, while Southern City policy makers and service providers had taken active steps toward providing sex education in the schools. Overwhelming support for schools to offer sex education has been documented in these two communities and among the state- and national-level participants in our study.

Nevertheless, gaps obviously exist. Policy makers, service providers, and the general public in both Farmville and Southern City were overwhelmingly in favor of the school systems' providing sex education and family life education in the classroom. Yet in Farmville 96 percent of the need for sex education at the high school level and 98 percent of the need for sex education at the junior high level was unmet. In Southern City, at the very best, 60 percent of the need for sex and family life education in the schools was unmet, and we suspect that, using our definition, an 80 percent unmet need in the Southern City school system would be a more realistic estimate. Why was there a nearly 100 percent unmet need in Farmville and between 60 and 80 percent in Southern City?

The answer does not lie in value gaps among the public, the service providers, and the policy makers. There is a consensus that sex education is an appropriate and desired activity for the public school system. There are many aspects to any answer regarding why, when such a clear majority of the public, the service providers, and the policy makers approve, so little is happening. We suspect the main problem is that the elected officials and the school boards and administrators do not understand the nature of the support they would have if they were to develop adequate sex education programs for their school systems. We are still at the stage in which a relatively small number of individuals publicly oppose sex education in the schools and can bring sex education programs to a halt because the school administrators and school board members have so little confidence in the level of support for sex education in the schools. Our study results indicate the presence of a mandate for the schools in these two communities to develop adequate sex education programs.

In this and the preceding chapters, we have examined the efforts to manage pregnancy and pregnancy prevention through contraceptive care and sex education in Farmville and Southern City. We asked the policy makers, service providers, general public, and teenage mothers in both communities what recommendations, if any, they had to help their community manage adolescent fertility more successfully. We turn in Chapter 9 to their recommendations and present our own conclusions.

9

RECOMMENDATIONS AND CONCLUSIONS

Tell every family in the county.
A Farmville county commissioner

What recommendations do the policy makers, service providers, and teenage mothers in these two communities have that might be useful to other communities concerned about the rate of pregnancies among their adolescents? To find out, we asked each person we interviewed whether he or she thought additional resources, changes, laws, or policies in relation to teenage pregnancies were needed in the community. If people thought no changes were needed, we asked them to tell us that. The respondents came up with an impressive and insightful number of recommendations. The directions and focuses of the recommendations varied with each individual's background and experiences. In order to allow the reader to judge the types of actions that each cluster of persons interviewed would recommend, we will provide a summary overview, then discuss each group in detail.

OVERVIEW OF RECOMMENDATIONS

A careful study of the action recommendations of policy makers (Table 9.1), service providers (Table 9.2), and teenagers (Table 9.3) in the two communities leads us to believe that knowledge of what to do to control teenage pregnancies already exists in both communities.

Recommendations from Farmville policy makers and service providers seemed to acknowledge that little was being done, and stated the need for action on numerous issues. Southern City policy makers'

TABLE 9.1

Summary of Policy Makers' Recommendations, Farmville and Southern City, 1977

Policy Makers	Issue	Action
Farmville		
County commissioners, city councilmen	Coordination	Coordinate agencies
	Communication	Set up communications networks
	Funding	Increase funding
	Public education	Provide sex education
	Multiagency effort	Involve all appropriate groups
Health board members	United Fund	United Fund support
	Churches	Church support
	County funds	County funding
	Civic clubs	Civic club support
	Private donors	Private donors
Named influentials	Liberal abortion	Liberalize abortion policies
	Early sex education	Teach sex education early and in depth
	Confidentiality	Guarantee agency confidentiality
	Counseling	Improve counseling
	Lower costs	Reduce costs of services to teenagers
	Publicity	Publicize available services
	Parent education	Educate parents
	Prevention	Fund pregnancy prevention programs
Social Services and Mental Health board members	Lead agency	Identify a lead agency
	Public recognition	Recognize the problem publicly

School board members	Health Department	Get more help from local Health Department
	Training counselors	Have trained counselors in junior and senior high schools
	Social workers	Hire social workers

Southern City

County commissioners	Family planning	Emphasize family planning
	Sex education	Improve sex education
	Quality of personnel	Secure higher-quality teachers and service providers
	Public health nurse	Assign a public health nurse to the school
	Public attitudes	Liberalize the public's attitude toward teenage pregnancy
Board of health	Laws	Liberalize the laws and policies concerning problem pregnancies
	Sex education	Improve sex education in the schools
	Funding	Assure adequate program funding
	Teen education	Inform teenage population
	Provider training	Train service providers
Social Services and Mental Health board members	Earlier sex education	Have sex education from the fourth grade through high school
	Communication	Improve communications at all levels
	Family planning services	Provide comprehensive family planning services in the schools
	Male involvement	Involve teenage male
	Approaches to problem	Use nontraditional approaches
School board members	Resources	Expand resources
	Policies	Liberalize school and agency policies
	Funding	Increase funding for pregnancy prevention programs
	Scope of effort	Focus on communitywide efforts
	Sex education	Provide more thorough sex education

Source: Compiled by the author.

TABLE 9.2

Summary of Service Providers' Recommendations, Farmville and Southern City, 1977

Service Providers	Issue	Action
Farmville		
Health Department staff	Clientele	Open Health Department to more women in need of family planning services
	Nurse practitioners	Staff additional family planning clinics with nurse practitioners
	Counselors	Hire additional staff to counsel and educate
	Family planning clinic	Have clinics devoted exclusively to family planning
	Full-time nurses	Employ full-time family planning nurses
	Physician time	Budget more physician time
	Prenatal care	Provide better prenatal care
	Funds	Provide more funds for public information
	In-service education	Allow nursing staff to get in-service education
	Abortion funds	Provide funds for abortion
Physicians	Action council	Form an action council
Pharmacists	Contraceptive availability	Make contraceptives more available
	Government assistance	Provide enough governmental assistance to make birth control accessible to everyone
	Counseling	Provide better counseling and sex education
Social workers	Barriers	Remove barriers to services for teenagers
	Sex education	Increase amount of sex education in the schools
Mental health workers	Coordination	Encourage interagency coordination
	Services	Increase services available to teenagers

Group	Topic	Recommendation
School administrators and counselors	Funds	Provide more funds to develop programs
	Hotline	Provide a hotline
	Listing	Develop a comprehensive listing of agencies and resources
Southern City		
Health Department staff	Early detection	Provide early detection of teenage pregnancy
	Resources	Expand available resources
Physicians	Sex education	Improve and expand sex education programs
	Support	Strengthen support for Health Department's efforts
	Laws	Liberalize laws and policies surrounding birth control
Pharmacists	Awareness	Increase public awareness of services available
	Sex education	Increase sex education at junior high level, emphasizing services available
	Center	Provide a low-profile center for education and services
Social and mental health workers	Barriers	Remove barriers to birth control services
	Sex education	Provide more sex education in the schools
	Resources	Commit county resources to a comprehensive pregnancy prevention program for teenagers
School administrators	Public action	Let the public start doing its share—then the schools will do theirs

Source: Compiled by the author.

TABLE 9.3

Summary of What Teenage Mothers State as Their Fertility-Related
Needs, Farmville and Southern City, 1977

Issue	Teenagers' Needs
Prevention	Knowledge of how to prevent pregnancy
Counseling	Someone to talk to
Costs	Access to free or low-cost contraceptives
Safety	Pills that do not cause cancer
Male education	Partner's early awareness of whether the girl is using birth control
Prenatal care	Better prenatal care
Child care skills	Information on how to care for children
Anger	Help in dealing with anger about pregnancy

Source: Compiled by the author.

and service providers' recommendations seemed to acknowledge that
an effort was under way, but called for numerous additional actions.

The recommendations are not easily categorized. Some of the
most constantly recurring themes were the need for better sex education and the provision of free birth control counseling and services
to all teenagers in the community. If the recommendations were to
be acted on as a group in both communities, we believe that the major
steps necessary to manage teenage pregnancies would have been taken.

The needs stated by the teenage mothers are addressed in the
policy makers' and service providers' recommendations. Teenagers
would be provided pregnancy prevention education, adequate counseling, access to free services, better prenatal care, and education in
infant care. The teenagers also asked for the young men involved to
share responsibility, safer contraceptives, and help in coping with
their anger over being pregnant. The sex education efforts called for
by the policy makers and service providers should lead to young men's
assuming more responsibility for pregnancy prevention. With increased contraceptive counseling, teenage girls in the two communities
could use the safer preventive methods (such as diaphragm and foam).
Greater success in preventing pregnancies will eliminate the anger
these teenagers report feeling when they discover they are uninten-
tionally pregnant.

We turn now to a detailed discussion of the recommendations of each group in the two communities.

FARMVILLE POLICY MAKERS

County Commissioners and City Councilmen

> Sex education in the schools, definitely.
> A Farmville county commissioner

Recommendations by the elected officials who control the policies and budgets within Farmville fell into five areas:

Coordinate the agencies,
Set up communications networks,
Increase funding,
Provide sex education in the public schools, and
Involve all appropriate groups.

Ten of the eleven county commissioners and city councilmen interviewed recommended changes. One city councilman said no changes seemed to be needed. All but one of the commissioners and councilmen were interviewed.

Coordinate Agencies

One commissioner suggested coordinating the agencies within Farmville that have any responsibilities for helping the community assist teenagers in managing their sexuality. Coordinating mental health and social services was specifically recommended. Another suggested that the local technical institute develop a program to ensure that all teenage parents earn a high school diploma.

Establish Communications Networks

It was in the second area, setting up communications networks, that the majority of recommendations came. Several commissioners recognized that they had little knowledge of the actual adolescent sexuality situation in Farmville, and felt that a publicity campaign was needed to "tell every family in the county." One speculated that most families in the county, like his own, did not know what services were available or what steps a teenager could take when she suspected she was pregnant. The commissioners spoke of needing "more ways of providing information to girls and boys about how to prevent pregnancy." Any communications network set up, a county commissioner concluded, should include "repeated discussions of human sexuality in all of the black churches and the poorer white churches." One commissioner recommended that many opportunities for sexually active adolescents to communicate their needs should be provided, observing that if the numbers of teenagers involved in the situation were known, one could "move mountains."

Increase Funding

Two of the commissioners focused on funding. One said, "If an organization was set up to handle the problem of teenage pregnancies, I would support changes they asked for." The strategy recommended was to seek federal funds first, but failing that, or in the interim, to fund a program to manage pregnancies among adolescents through an existing agency.

Give Additional Attention to Sex Education

Public education and sex education efforts clearly needed attention, in the minds of Farmville's elected policy makers. One called for a public awareness campaign so that local citizens would know where to go and what was available. Commissioners and councilmen seemed impatient with the sex education efforts in the schools. Their language was strong. After calling for sex education for the parents as well as the teenagers, one commissioner added, "Sex education in the schools, definitely." Other commissioners and councilmen were even more emphatic. One wanted to see earlier sex education. He recommended that while it might be voluntary in the elementary schools, sex education should be "mandatory in high school." A city councilman insisted that sex education begin in the first grade, using what he termed a "scientific approach." He felt that the state government must insist on an integrated sex education program. "An integrated program (beginning in the first grade) needs to be forced from the state or federal [level]," he concluded.

The Farmville county commissioners and city councilmen, with the exception of the one councilman already noted, all had recommendations for varying types of action. The overall impression was that these officials were receptive to efforts to manage adolescent fertility in Farmville better, and were impatient with the slowness with which the community agencies and groups were responding.

Increase the Number of Groups Involved

The commissioners and councilmen recommended a number of agencies and groups that they thought should be concerned. In addition to the Health Department, social services, and the mental health center, churches and civic organizations were mentioned. The chamber of commerce was frequently mentioned as a concerned group, and the Junior Women's League and the Jayceettes were named. Individuals mentioned were doctors in private practice and their nurses. One official said he knew some of the clergy were interested in the level of problem pregnancies among the local teenagers.

Board of Health

As mentioned earlier, Farmville has a five-county Health Department and board of health unit. The Farmville member of the board of health whom we were able to interview responded enthusiastically, outlining a five-point approach he felt should be made: (1) United Fund support, (2) church support, (3) county funds, (4) civic club support, and (5) private donors.

First, he explained, a strong United Fund exists in Farmville. The board member felt the Executive Committee of the United Fund, of which he was a member, would be interested in providing funds to improve adolescent fertility management. Second, he believed the churches would be willing to help through a number of in-kind contributions, such as office help, typing, and counseling services. Third, he thought the county commissioners would be willing to appropriate certain funds and would view such a project as good. Fourth, the civic clubs in Farmville had a council with members from every organization. He believed the civic clubs would view a program aimed at improved management of adolescent pregnancy as a good cause. Finally, the board member believed there were private donors throughout the county who would be interested in contributing money to the effort.

It is not possible to know to what extent each of these groups and individuals would actually contribute time and money to assist the county in developing a program to deal with excess fertility among adolescents. However, this community leader was frequently mentioned when we asked each participant to name the two or three most influential persons in the county who might be concerned about problem pregnancies among the teenagers. That he believed all these supportive events to be easily possible indicated that he perceived the atmosphere in the community to be receptive.

Other Named Influentials

The ten named Farmville influentials we interviewed, in addition to the health board member described above, tended to make practical, programmatically oriented recommendations: liberalize abortion policies further, teach sex education early and in depth, guarantee agency confidentiality, improve counseling, reduce costs of services to teenagers, publicize available services, educate the parents, and fund pregnancy prevention programs.

Nine of the ten felt that new policies and programs were needed; one said he was not sure. Those interviewed included ministers, the head of the chamber of commerce, a top bank official, the head of the local branch of the National Association for the Advancement of Colored People, and several teachers in the local schools. One named influential felt that Farmville needed a policy favoring abortion that could be made known in the schools and in the community. He also said, "Sex education needs to be taught in the schools early and heavy—ten-year-olds need to know the dangerous parts." He favored having one agency to which teenagers could turn and be guaranteed confidentiality. If such an agency did not exist, he believed younger teenagers would not go anywhere and their pregnancies would not be discovered until their mothers became suspicious.

Three of the influentials emphasized a need for in-depth counseling. One said specifically that Farmville needed a "better counseling system to let teenagers know they are loved and cared for. More positive counseling . . . to prevent teenage pregnancies . . . more in-depth, sincere counseling." One named influential specifically saw a need for more cooperation among "the Health Department, Department of Social Services, and the school principals."

Reducing the costs of services that teenagers must pay for was mentioned along with "publicizing the availability of services." The respondents felt that what could already be done in Farmville was not made public. One named influential felt it as important to educate and counsel the parents as the teens. He emphasized that while he felt the teen already pregnant needs help, he would prefer to see any funding go toward education and prevention of problem pregnancies.

The general impression left by the named influentials with whom we had interviews was that they felt a need for policies to be developed in the community, for greater confidentiality, for improvements in the type and level of counseling being done in the community, and for cooperation among the Health Department, social services, and mental health personnel. Their responses conveyed a sense that little was being done, and a feeling on their part that much needed to be done. The basic feeling communicated by the named influentials was concern about the teenage pregnancy problem and a feeling that the community needed to respond more sensitively to teenagers' needs for confidentiality and supportive counseling.

The Social Services and Mental Health Boards

Members of the Farmville social services and mental health boards were similarly action-oriented in their program recommendations: identify a lead agency and recognize the problem publicly. The social services board members favored identifying a lead agency. "One agency should be identified to handle problem pregnancies, and that agency should be well known—the Health Department would be the logical agency," commented one social services board member.

Recommendations by the mental health board members were similar. One member said there "should be a designated agency for pregnancy services coordination." Another called for "program planning and coordination," saying that public policy should be based on a philosophy of recognizing needs. Another member concluded, "If agencies need more money for programs, they should get it. People should come out and recognize the problem publicly."

School Board

> Adolescent pregnancy has low priority in the county
> . . . the information level is spotty.
>
> A school board member

School board members seemed not to have thought as much about the problem of unintended teenage pregnancies in Farmville as had members of the boards of mental health and social services. One school board member commented, "The school board really isn't concerned about it [pregnancies among teenagers] and I think it is something we really ought to do . . . I detect a fatalistic attitude." Pregnancies among teenagers should not be of particular concern to the school board, according to one member. Another member said he was not prepared to comment on whether he would recommend any changes in the current situation in Farmville schools.

Other school board members were somewhat more concerned. Three suggestions emerged: (1) get more help from the local Health Department, (2) have trained counselors in the junior and senior high schools, and (3) hire social workers. One board member wanted "more help from the local Health Department." Another saw a need for "resources for counseling in high school and junior high. We need a counselor whose expertise is particular to the problem of adolescent pregnancies." Another board member called for more information in the schools and "more social workers to help pregnant girls." He explained that such counselors should be designated and advertised in the schools so that girls would know of the availability of help. The board member concluded by saying that the Health Department was the logical place to get help for the pregnancy problem in the schools.

The two other school board members were pessimistic about school board involvement. One commented, "No system of care has emerged in the county so far—it looks like the best situation is to be an AFDC mother's daughter." (These daughters have a social worker taking a direct interest in their welfare, including any problem pregnancies that may occur.) Concerning the possibility that the counselors presently in the school system can help teenage girls with fertility control problems, the member commented, "I truthfully do not believe our school counselors have the kind of relationship that kind of thing requires."

The last school board member we interviewed observed that originally the teenage pregnancy problem was among blacks from lower socioeconomic groups, but nobody was safe from it now. It covered the whole spectrum of students. He said, "The schools need sex education, but we [the board] have taken the stance that nothing can be done about it." He said he felt that while the problem of unintended pregnancies could not be eliminated entirely, something could be done. "I think the thing contributing most to the problem is this attitude that nothing can be done."

SOUTHERN CITY POLICY MAKERS

County Commissioners

Southern City county commissioners leaned toward five policies: (1) emphasize family planning, (2) improve sex education, (3) secure higher-quality teachers and service providers, (4) assign a public health nurse to the schools, and (5) change the public's attitudes about teenage pregnancy.

Among the three Southern City county commissioners we were able to interview, feelings ran from "We're doing a good job already" to a felt need for doing more. When asked what, if any, changes were needed, one commissioner responded, "No changes are needed; we're really pretty well organized. There is an emphasis on family planning which has been very commendable. The laws are not prohibitive." In fact, the laws at the time did prohibit providing birth control to minors without parental consent, but the Health Department and the county commissioners felt the need among teenagers was too compelling to ignore. The second county commissioner felt action was needed to provide more sex education in the school system.

The third county commissioner had five recommendations:

Sex education should be better presented and taught with parental
knowledge.
Quality persons with preparation and appropriate attitudes should
teach and provide services.
The service capacity of the Southern City Health Department should
be increased.
A public health nurse, "a person of high caliber," should be assigned
to the schools.
The attitudes of the people should be changed along with provision of
services.

Specifically, he felt that the attitudes of doctors and nurses
needed to improve; presumably he meant that they should be more
sympathetic to problems faced by teenagers with unintended pregnancies.

Board of Health

Southern City health board member attitudes covered a wide
range of opinions: rethink the laws and policies concerning problem
pregnancies, improve sex education in the schools, assure adequate
program funding, inform the teenage population, and train the service
providers. Two board members focused on provision of services.
One was anxious to "make sure available programs are adequately
funded to provide services." Another member recommended a coordinated effort to disseminate information to the target population,
funds to finance it, and proper training for service providers. Three
had no specific recommendations to make.

Departments of Social Services and Mental Health

Recommendations from the two members of the Department of
Social Services identified as the most informed on the subject of teen
pregnancies differed widely: one was not sure what to recommend,
and the other had some very definite ideas about what Southern City
ought to be doing in the area of managing adolescent fertility: have
sex education from the fourth grade through high school, improve
communication at all levels, provide comprehensive family planning
services in the schools, involve the teenage male, and use nontraditional approaches. The second board member felt that "sex education
can be taught in an inoffensive manner, dwelling more on prevention
of pregnancy than anatomy." In addition, she advocated "finding out
about each child's background. We need to go deeper into why the girls

get pregnant by examining home, community, church, school and parental attitudes. "

Mental health board members had several suggestions to make. One wanted to see a "policy that would temporarily suspend a pregnant child from school at a time predetermined by the Board of Education with provision to return." Having said this, he stated that communication at the levels of home and agencies was not sufficient. He said there was a need in Southern City for "more coordination of services." He liked the idea of one agency's being responsible, with "subagency cooperation," then concluded, "Someone has to call the shots."

Another member made several recommendations. She said, "The Southern City schools do not make comprehensive services available to students." She felt that comprehensive family planning services should be made available in the schools. She states, "There is apparently a lack of resources in terms of counseling." Further, "Most programs only relate to females. Let's look at the teenage males question! Nontraditional approaches to getting at the youths and providing information are needed. Schools cannot bear the entire burden for social/moral questions."

School Board

School board members' responses to the question about whether changes are needed were varied. Two of the ten board members had no recommendations; two others said no changes were needed. The remaining six had some recommendations they would like to see implemented: expand the resources, improve school and agency policies, increase funding for pregnancy prevention programs, focus on communitywide efforts, and provide more thorough sex education.

Three members had action-oriented recommendations to make. One advocated "increasing general knowledge in the community about what is involved." She added, "The school system is neglected. They try, but funding and community attitudes are negative about their involvement." A second board member wanted to see "counseling and dissemination of information through agencies that really reach young people. Not two or three agencies, but community-wide efforts need to be made, including involving responsible board members." The final member of the school board recommended more "sex education including emotional and functional elements, counseling services on abortion, prenatal and postnatal care and parenting training."

Board members in both communities were involved and wanted to see numerous changes. On the whole, the board members in Southern City seemed to have thought more about the issue of managing adolescent fertility in their community, and so had more recommendations to make than Farmville board members. Aside from a few members in both communities who had no changes to recommend, there was support for more community action among all of the board members who participated in the study. We encountered no identifiable opposition to the schools' or other public agencies' or groups' becoming more involved in managing adolescent fertility in the two communities.

FARMVILLE SERVICE PROVIDERS

Health Department Staff

> There is no place in Farmville offering counseling to teenagers with problem pregnancies.
>> A Health Department
>> family planning nurse

The Health Department staff had a significant number of recommendations for improvements in the Health Department:

Open the Health Department clinic to more people and have nurses trained as maternal health practitioners—that is, break the bottleneck of insufficient physician resources by having the nurse practitioners see the family planning patients on clinic days;
Make more staff available for counseling and education;
Have clinics devoted exclusively to family planning;
Employ nurses who devote full time to family planning;
Budget more physician time;
Get a physician with whom the staff can communicate;
Provide better prenatal care (present care is characterized by long waits, no doctors, no back-up, and no nutritionist, according to staff members);
Provide more money to the Health Department for public information;
Allow the nursing staff to get continuing in-service education; and
Provide money for abortions.

Several Health Department staff members mentioned a need for better sex education in the schools and in the community, but their major focus was on improving the services at the Health Department itself. They were intensely dissatisfied with the small number of family planning patients being seen each week, and were concerned with finding ways to provide full-time family planning staff and additional funding to accommodate the women currently being turned away each week.

Physicians

Of the eight key physicians with whom we had interviews, four saw no special problems within Farmville in the area of pregnancies among schoolgirls, and felt no changes were really necessary. The other four, however, were disturbed by the level of pregnancies among teenagers in Farmville, and recommended the formation of a board with representatives from the schools, social services, public health, the Ministerial Association, and the medical society to make plans for improved community management of adolescent fertility. They indicated that they did not feel that an entire agency was needed for these purposes. Rather, they advocated an action council consisting at least of representatives from the groups named.

Pharmacists

There are them that do . . . them that won't tell . . . but all do.

A Farmville pharmacist

Pharmacists in Farmville had a rather large number of recommendations for changes they felt were needed to achieve better community management of the fertility level among teenagers. Their recommendations clustered around three general approaches: (1) make contraceptives more available, (2) provide governmental assistance and total accessibility to birth control for everyone, and (3) provide better counseling and sex education.

One pharmacist had several recommendations: "Contraceptives should be available for the asking. The poor in Farmville should be given contraceptives free. Condoms should be sold at cost. Birth control devices need to be readily available to people without embarrassment." He also wanted the community to provide as much information as possible on fertility control.

The second area of recommendations from Farmville pharmacists was governmental assistance to persons wanting birth control supplies and counseling. One pharmacist insisted on the designation of one agency to coordinate federal, state, and county funding. His goal for Farmville was "total accessibility" to birth control for everyone in the community.

All of the Farmville pharmacists emphasized the existence of a strong need in the community for better counseling help for teenagers.

They wanted to see informal "rap sessions" and were eager to have more sex education in the high school.

What was impressive about the Farmville pharmacists' responses was their consistent reference to the presence of unacceptably low levels of access to contraceptives and of information and sex education for teenagers in the community.

These pharmacists appeared to be relied upon heavily for sex education and birth control information. Beyond the need for education and information, the pharmacists reflected strong concern about the apparent inability of teenagers and the poor in the community to buy contraceptives. The need for free contraceptives for the poor (and they seemed to include most Farmville teenagers in this category) had made a strong enough impression on the pharmacists for them to advocate making available free a line of items that normally brings good profits to drugstores.

Social and Mental Health Workers

School is home away from home.
A Farmville social worker

All Farmville social workers made recommendations for changes. These focused on two areas of concern: (1) remove the barriers to services for teenagers and (2) increase the amount of sex education in the schools.

In the area of removal of barriers, social workers emphasized allowing teenagers access to contraceptives, abortion, and pregnancy tests without parental consent. In the area of sex education, they emphasized involving community groups such as the Parent Teachers Association in holding conferences at which parents and teenagers could develop better rapport in the area of adolescent sexuality. The social workers recommended better coordination of community agencies, more information for the public and the teenagers, and a widespread literature distribution system. Generally they were emphatic about providing sex education in the schools. As one put it, "Sex education should be required at an early stage—fourth grade." One social worker stated that, in her view, "Sex education in schools should be mandatory" and that "a birth control distribution system should be mandatory."

Workers at the Mental Health Department focused their recommendations on two points: (1) encourage interagency coordination and (2) increase services available to teenagers. One mental health worker had a very specific proposal: "Hire four public health nurses to develop a pregnancy program. They would be responsible for picking

up all pregnancies among teens and working along with a private medical doctor." She, like most of the Farmville social workers, had
given up on the Public Health Department.

School Administrators and Counselors

School personnel focused on three suggestions: (1) provide more
money to develop programs, (2) have a hotline, and (3) develop a
comprehensive listing of agencies and resources. Among the 15 school
administrators and counselors interviewed, the most consistent recommendation was for money for the schools to develop programmatic
responses to the high incidence of unplanned teenage pregnancies.
One administrator emphasized the need for a hot line: "If they could
simply pick up a phone and talk over alternatives." Another recommended developing a "comprehensive listing of agencies and resources." Several administrators mentioned a need for pregnancy
prevention but, interestingly enough, only one mentioned a need for
early sex education.

SOUTHERN CITY SERVICE PROVIDERS

Health Department Staff

> Sex education is only the tip of the iceberg—more em-
> phasis should be placed on the long-term consequences,
> for example, the societal costs of adolescent pregnancies.
> A Southern City
> family planning worker

Health Department personnel recommended two basic directions:
(1) provide for early detection of teenage pregnancy and (2) expand the
available resources. Staff workers at the Southern City Health Department emphasized early detection: "some way to get them [teens
who have just discovered they are pregnant] across the fantasy border
before the pregnancy becomes advanced." Some mentioned a need for
more resources.
The overall impression, however, was that these recommendations were not focused on needs for changes within the Health Department family planning program. In our opinion this reveals a high
level of satisfaction among the family planning staff with both the way
the family planning clinics were being operated and the policies and
practices followed.

Physicians

> Too many resources now.
>> A Southern City physician

Of the 14 physicians in Southern City who were identified as key persons in the area of family planning and who participated in our study, 4 said no changes were needed, one commenting that there were "too many resources now." The other 10 physicians offered recommendations focused primarily on the following ideas: improve and expand sex education programs, strengthen support of the Health Department's efforts, and change the laws and policies on birth control.

One physician recommended "a widespread educational effort." Other recommendations were similar to that of one pediatrician: "Education—more people need to be more knowledgeable about what is here [in Southern City] and why it is important. Schools should take a more active role in teaching family life and responsible parenthood." A gynecologist at the Southern City Medical Center wanted what must be considered very early sex education. His recommendation was to "get sex education in the public schools by age five."

The high support level for the Public Health Department noted earlier among these physicians continued to be evident. One recommended that Southern City "strengthen support for the Health Department program and the ob-gyn clinic at the county hospital."

Several of the physicians recommended changing the laws. One wanted the state to change the law to let nonphysicians provide contraceptives to teenagers. One expressed concern that "U.S. federal government rulings lack consistency and negate state efforts." Another physician said he was concerned about the cutoff of federal funds for low-income persons needing fertility control assistance (abortions). In sum, Southern City physicians who participated in the study were supportive of the Health Department clinic efforts, wanted more sex education in the schools, and favored relaxing policies that allowed contraceptives to be prescribed only by licensed medical doctors.

Pharmacists

> ADVERTISE—make services known.
>> A Southern City pharmacist

Pharmacists' recommendations in Southern City reflected the intense concern with the lack of information among teenagers already seen in Farmville pharmacists' recommendations. Only five pharmacists were interviewed, but the recommendations from all five were similar: increase the public's awareness of the available services, increase sex education at the junior high level, especially emphasizing services available, and take action to plan a "low-profile" service center, to provide education and services.

Social Workers

> Needed: an understanding, sympathetic, empathetic system.
>
> A Southern City social worker

Recommendations of Southern City social workers were similar to those of the social workers in Farmville. They focused primarily on three points: (1) remove barriers to birth control services for teenagers, (2) provide more sex education in the schools, and (3) commit county resources to a comprehensive pregnancy prevention program for teenagers.

Among the eight social workers who participated in the study, only one felt that no changes were needed. Several of the social workers had strong views. One wanted to change the entire clinic system, give more sex education in the schools, and change parents' attitudes. Another social worker was emphatic about program needs, and recommended that "county officials [the elected leadership] recognize the problem and commit themselves to a comprehensive program utilizing all county resources. The school system," she added, "has the attitude 'throw them out.' Officials' attitudes generally need improvement." A third social worker concluded that the strongest need was for "an understanding, empathetic system."

School Administrators

> Educate the public to try to deal with the problem.
>
> A Southern City counselor

> Inform kids earlier of the consequences of teenage pregnancy.
>
> A Southern City
> school administrator

The recommendations of the 11 Southern City school principals and 3 school counselors were remarkable for what they did not recommend. One dominant theme emerged: let the public start doing its share—then the schools will do theirs.

Of the 14 principals and counselors interviewed, only one made any reference to improving sex education in the schools. The school principals saw the public as derelict in its responsibilities to provide better communication and sex education to the youth in the community. Their recommendations left the public schools strategically unmentioned. Instead, they spoke of "availability of services in terms of contraceptives" and "some group that would be in closer contact with the schools," "adult education," and "public awareness programs for adults and parents in community to assist with problems of teenagers."

These responses do not indicate that the school administrators and counselors were opposed to schools' doing their share of sex education. The overwhelming message conveyed, however, is that these respondents wanted the public and other agencies to assume a much larger share of responsibility for the sex education of community youth and provision of birth control measures to sexually active teenagers.

TEENAGERS' RECOMMENDATIONS

> Guys need family planning. I don't think they realize the trouble they can cause.
>
> A teenage girl

The teenagers interviewed were more vocal when it came to making recommendations for change. The interviewer asked each teenager the following question: "If you were asked to help design a program to help meet the needs of teenagers in the area of family planning, pregnancy, and child care, what things would you suggest?" While the question was deliberately open ended, the answers were not. Teens said they need the following:

Knowledge about how to prevent pregnancy,
Someone to talk to,
Access to free or low-cost contraceptives,
Pills that do not cause cancer,
Partner's early awareness of whether the other is using birth control,
Better prenatal care,
Information on how to care for children, and
Help in dealing with anger about pregnancy.

Martha Maxwell told the interviewer, "People mostly tell you stuff to scare you, not to help you. They hurt real bad. It would be much better if they would explain things—things they could use to prevent pregnancy."

Pregnancy Prevention

The comments made by the girls generally followed the three categories representing their areas of greatest concern. The first of these concerned pregnancy prevention and learning about and having access to appropriate contraceptive methods before becoming pregnant. By and large, girls indicated that there was no place to go to talk and no one to talk to, and that most of the information they did acquire came from friends and peers. Farmville girls acknowledged that they had learned some "facts of life" at school.

The teaching of the biology of sex in a biology class provides a Catch-22 situation for all involved. The biology teacher is charged with teaching the subject matter, but not with dealing with the emotions or the psychological aspects of sex. The students are eager to learn. Certainly they need to know the biology of sex, but without a psychological component and some means of coping with their often intense emotions, there is little benefit to them in simply knowing the biology. "They teach us well, and all that, but you know there is still something missing," Jessica Davis told the interviewer. One teen recommended that a sex education course be taught at the Department of Social Services or somewhere else in the community.

Opinions differed as to whether young men should be included in the classes. Several girls felt that the fellows did not care, and that there was no point in including them because they would not attend anyway. Others felt that it would be good to include the young men and make them feel somewhat more responsible for their actions. Winnie Simms, a 17-year-old mother, added, "Guys usually have sex around six times before they will even ask if the girl is taking anything."

Attempts to obtain contraceptives when they were needed often resulted in failure. Francine Jones had tried to get contraceptives at the Health Department. She was told that she needed her mother's signature in order to receive the prescription for the pill. Francine told the interviewer she knew she could not ask her mother for her signature because her mother thought "I was the sweetest little thing." The girl could have lied, but she knew that was wrong. Since she knew of no other options, she became a teenage mother.

With respect to family planning, a number of girls indicated a desire to have good family planning clinics for young people. They indicated that access to contraceptive information was fairly limited and that they needed more information before they could choose the type of contraceptive that would be best for them. Many girls thought of the pill as synonymous with contraception, but a number of them were afraid to take it because they believed that it caused cancer. Olive Rogers spoke for many girls when she said, "Haven't you seen those ads on television where they tell you the pills cause cancer? I'm not taking them." Some girls felt that any program needed to go beyond simply providing information. A number thought that all girls should be cautioned on the risks they were taking when they became sexually active. "It's dumb to get pregnant if you don't want the baby," summarized one Southern City teenager. There was also a feeling that the cost of contraception should not be prohibitive. Money seemed to be one of the major concerns of teens in making recommendations for potential programs.

Preparation for Parenthood

Bodily changes, both emotional and physical, during pregnancy, labor, and delivery were the specific issues that constituted the second area of concern. As far as could be determined, there were no Lamaze, Bradley, or other types of classes to prepare women for labor and delivery available in Farmville. Therefore, only those girls who went on a tour of the county hospital had any notion of what to expect of their pregnancy or delivery.

The item suggested most often by teenagers was to show films about pregnancy and childbearing. Girls felt that the films should be shown to both young men and young women, so that the men might have a better idea of what their partners were going through.

Not all teens agreed that it would make their partners more responsible, but they all agreed that it was worth a try. A second often-voiced suggestion was to provide counseling—to have someone talk to you, to share your thoughts, feelings, and fears of pregnancy and delivery. Most pregnant teens got only two types of information about the process of delivery. From their mothers they heard, "You will get through it." From friends who had already had babies, they heard exaggerated tales of what it was really like. Both types of information served to make the girl about to go through delivery even more uncertain and anxious, and neither provided her with any facts.

Concern for the Newborn

The responsibility of caring for a child when one is barely past childhood oneself is something that few teenagers anticipate. Concern for the child immediately after birth and during the toddler years formed the third focus of concern. One Farmville teen said that she wished there was a place teens could go to learn about how to care for children and how to know when they were sick and when they were not. One teenager in Southern City was able to go to a single parents' course sponsored by the Health Department. Though that particular group consisted mostly of older persons, she was able to anticipate some of the events that were soon to be happening to her, and was able to derive a certain amount of support for her new life-style from these people. She eventually formed her own club for single parents and asked a number of people her own age to join. The club's purpose was to discuss the girls' problems with people that they knew.

There were concerns, too, about the male's role in the situation. The previous year most of these males were little more than young boys having some fun. Now they were fathers, but not husbands, and they were less sure than the girls about what to do in their new role. One Southern City girl suggested that their partners, boyfriends, or even former boyfriends should be included in any counseling or discussions. Such assistance, she thought, would help the men to clarify their role and what should be expected of that role, whether or not they were still seeing their child's mother regularly. The girl also felt that such an arrangement would help girls like herself to feel less angry. For those who were able to talk things out and share the responsibility of the child, in both time and money, the adjustment to early motherhood seemed considerably easier. However, such couples were the exception rather than the rule, for neither Farmville nor Southern City had chosen to focus its concern or services on meeting the needs of these child parents.

EFFECTS OF THE TWO
ORGANIZATIONAL APPROACHES

We have examined many externally measurable results of the approaches to managing adolescent fertility taken by two communities. We believe much can be learned for future programmatic decision making by analytically examining the approaches to family planning and prenatal care in the two communities. In both communities the Public Health Department was the agency providing the community organizational effort to manage teenage pregnancies. As we have seen, the two departments filled this role very differently. These behavioral differences led to important consequences that we have measured in the first eight chapters. We focus now on the differences and their results.

Approaches to Defining Organizational Policies

Farmville: Operate within established guidelines.
Southern City: Focus on making services available.

The basic policy of the Farmville Health Department was to operate only within established guidelines set by state laws, by federal laws and regulations, and by the county commissioners. Guidelines for approaching the management of pregnancies among adolescents in the community also came from the overall policies of the agency itself. Agency policies were in part reflections of what the agency believed about itself (its self-image) and its perceptions of the community within which it operated.

The basic orientation of the Farmville Health Department was to the policies and regulations determined by various others. In contrast, the Southern City Health Department approach was to emphasize availability of services rather than the following of regulations. The orientation that shaped the policies and service decisions of the Southern City Health Department was identifying community health needs, then providing services to all who asked for them. The Southern City Health Department took into account established guidelines set by state and federal laws, but it did not allow itself to be defined by them. The department did not take lightly the policies set by the county commissioners and its own political perception of the community within which it operated; neither did it allow itself to be fully defined by local perception.

The Farmville Health Department also sought to identify community health needs, then to provide services to the public. However, it was the basic organizational orientation of these two departments that led to major differences in their behaviors. For example, both were concerned about the large number of problem pregnancies occurring among teenagers each year. However, when the Farmville Health Department shaped its basic response to the perceived needs, the externally existing policies and regulations played the major role in determining how the department responded. In the approach taken by the Southern City Health Department, policies and guidelines were blended with needs for service availability as the primary consideration. The importance of the influences of these two differing organizational orientations can be illustrated in several ways.

Organizational Self-Image

Farmville: Fill only the gaps left by private medical practitioners.
Southern City: Define the task, then convince the community.

The family planning programs of the Farmville and Southern City Health Departments were profoundly affected by the past histories of the two agencies. The Farmville family planning program grew out of the prenatal care program begun in 1962 by Farmville physicians to reduce the number of welfare mothers coming to their private offices. Thus, in the area of prenatal care, as in other areas of health care, the role defined for the Farmville Health Department over the years was to fill the gaps left by private medical practitioners. In short, the areas permitted the Health Department were whatever areas the private physicians were not filling or did not intend to fill. The local physicians usually staffed clinics and other activities of the Farmville Health Department, making it in some sense an extension of their own practices. Thus the Farmville Health Department image was that of doing whatever the private medical community assigned to it or left otherwise unattended.

In contrast, the Southern City Health Department family planning program grew in a milieu of fierce independence. The Health Department's self-image was to move to meet identified needs in any way it could. Being in a larger community, the department enjoyed relatively greater independence from the local physicians. The staff first defined its own image, then set about making that image accepted in the professional community. While the basic sources of organizational self-understanding were external to the Farmville Health Department, they were internal to that of Southern City. This characteristic was manifested in their funding approaches, rules for deciding on risk taking, and leadership concepts.

Funding Approaches

Farmville: The county cannot help.
Southern City: Only county help is needed.

The funding approach used in the Farmville Health Department was to establish a family planning program with federal and state financial assistance. Thus the impetus, and consequently the guidelines, for expenditures came from external sources. The Farmville Health Department assumed that the county commissioners could not or would not pay for family planning for county residents. In contrast, partly in order not to become encumbered by federal and state guidelines, the Southern City Health Department insisted that only local county funds be used for family planning. Its policy was to offer all family planning services free to any resident.

Risk Taking

Farmville: Do not take risks.
Southern City: Blend political feasibility and needs.

Prior funding decisions directly affected decisions on risk taking in the two Health Departments. The policy in Farmville was to operate within guidelines. Thus, following state guidelines, the Farmville Health Department insisted on parental consent for family planning services and required that the parent sign the consent form in the presence of a Health Department staff member. Following federal guidelines requiring greater local budget contributions each year, Farmville sent all persons seeking family planning services to be screened for Title 19 or Title 20 eligibility. In conformity with what Farmville Health Department policy makers perceived to be the preferred policies of the local physicians, they discouraged any resident who had a private physician from participating in the department's family planning program.

The Southern City approach to risk-taking behavior arose out of a blend of what seemed politically feasible and what community health service needs were believed to be. During a decade when most other family planning programs in the state refused to provide birth control to minors without parental consent, the Southern City family planning program served anyone who asked for birth control, regardless of age or marital status. The principle of maximum availability of services to residents took precedence over views of the state's lawyers, who said that while it was unlikely, the department could possibly be sued by parents whose minor children were treated without their consent. The staff at the Southern City Health Department decided it was worth risking a lawsuit in order to serve a population of teenagers in need of services. Service availability, not conformity to externally developed regulations, was the standard by which decisions involving risk were made. The clearest example of this standard was the decision that no family planning patient was ever asked to seek to qualify for Title 19 or Title 20 eligibility. The Southern City staff believed that this demeaned the patient and discouraged the use of the services.

Approaches to Leadership

Farmville: Leadership may be frowned upon.
Southern City: Leadership is expected.

What were the working assumptions about the appropriate role of a Health Department in helping a community develop strategies to reduce unintended pregnancies among teenagers? Following its historic experiences, the Farmville Health Department operated on the belief that leadership may be frowned upon by the local physicians, and perhaps by other important poeple in the community. In clear contrast, the Southern City Health Department assumed its leadership would be accepted and that it was expected to lead in identifying and providing services to teenagers in the community.

These two approaches to leadership have important implications for the major recommendation we make from this study. Here we refer to the "lead agency" concept as demonstrated by the behavior of these two public health agencies. In Farmville the Health Department believed it had no responsibilities beyond its organizationally defined roles. These organizational roles came from a number of sources, including state and federal regulations, county commissioners' policies, and informal perceptions of community preferences.

In Southern City the Public Health Department provided communitywide leadership in the effort to manage adolescent fertility more successfully. Operationally, this resulted in what was perceived by others to be a "lead agency" position for the Health Department. The Health Department staff operated on the assumption that the public policy makers, such as the county commissioners and the medical community, would accept leadership perceived as adequate and meeting a community need.

AUTHORS' RECOMMENDATIONS

In the introduction to this book, we stated that, in our view, sufficient birth control technology (however imperfect it may be) already exists to enable communities to reduce pregnancy rates drastically. We argued that what communities do to manage adolescent fertility depends less on technology and more on the social values among the general public, policy makers, and public service agencies. We believe that the recommendations for change made by the policy makers, service providers, and teenage mothers in the two communities demonstrate that the basic knowledge and ideas needed for more successful management of adolescent fertility already exist in Farmville and Southern City. It is not a lack of knowledge that is the key problem. Rather, it is the lack of leadership or a "lead agency." We believe the Southern City orientation to community management of adolescent fertility can serve as a powerful model for other communities concerned about the pregnancy rates among their teenagers.

The data in Chapters 3 through 8 show that a Southern City approach has impacts. Impacts can be achieved even without massive federal or state aid, and leadership by a "lead agency" such as the Health Department is accepted in this community. This approach does not require anything dramatic, but its achievements in making fertility services available to adolescents can be dramatic.

Initiatives in providing fertility control assistance to adolescents must be taken in each community. The impetus need not be from the

Public Health Department. However, in most communities the Health Department is already involved in providing fertility management help to community members. Adolescent fertility is already viewed as an appropriate and legitimate public health problem.

On the basis of the Southern City experience, we believe a successful approach to community management of teenage pregnancy rates will have at least the following identifiable characteristics:

A "lead (seriously concerned) agency" emerges;

Counseling, pregnancy tests, contraceptives, abortions, and prenatal care are made readily available to all teenagers;

As a result of "lead agency" efforts, an informal communications system emerges—professionals in agencies and physicians in private practice routinely refer teenagers to a community resource (usually a service in the Health Department) for counseling, pregnancy tests, contraceptives, abortion referral, and prenatal care services;

Schools create their own action policies and guidebooks to develop a school-based sex education program; and

The approach is person-centered.

In the final analysis, teenage pregnancy is a social-value issue. Southern City is committed to accepting the teenagers and responding to them as persons with needs that the community has an obligation to meet.

SUMMARY AND CONCLUSIONS

We have examined in great detail the efforts of two communities to manage fertility among their teenagers. In Farmville the efforts were focused on operating within established organizational guidelines. In Southern City they were focused on making fertility control services readily available to teenagers. Because of their more restrictive orientations, the agencies and residents of Farmville were having little success in their efforts to manage fertility among the adolescent population. Southern City had not finished the task, but the schools and the Health Department had begun a process that appeared to be leading to successful management of adolescent fertility in the community.

In conclusion, let us again focus on the four basic research questions we posed about the American Public Health Association (APHA) policies for communities to use to manage adolescent fertility more successfully.

The first question we sought to answer is, To what extent are the needs identified in the APHA policies already being met? In our opinion the citizens of Southern City had already moved significantly toward adopting most of the policies the APHA recommends. For example, adolescents in Southern City tended to be treated nonjudgmentally and as individuals. Southern City teenagers were being provided substantial access to sex education, contraceptives, pregnancy testing, abortion, and prenatal care without requiring parental consent. Except for the $3 pregnancy test fee, services were free. Efforts at early detection were being made in the local schools. All alternatives for dealing with the pregnancy were presented as acceptable solutions. A number of community agencies, including the Health, Social Services, and Mental Health Departments and the schools, were working to meet the needs of sexually active adolescents. We believe it can be reasonably concluded that efforts to assist sexually active adolescents in Southern City conformed substantially to the policies recommended by the APHA.

In contrast, the efforts in Farmville were in substantial nonconformity. Adolescents in Farmville were treated more judgmentally, and privacy and confidentiality were constantly mentioned as lacking by both service providers and teenage service recipients. Access to sex education, contraceptive services, and pregnancy testing was subject to several barriers not present in Southern City. Parental consent, for example, was required in Farmville. Because there were so many barriers to care, teenagers felt that support was lacking. Little was done to detect pregnancy in the early stages, and virtually no information was available in the schools or elsewhere in the community. Abortion, however, was readily available, as it was in Southern City. Again, however, there appeared to be more barriers to abortion services for Farmville teenagers. Finally, in Farmville no agency had taken active leadership in bringing the needs of sexually active teenagers to public attention or in organizing services that emphasized availability to the community's teenagers.

It was not the case that Southern City was meeting all of the APHA policy recommendations and Farmville none of them. Farmville, however, had made very little progress toward implementing the types of recommendations made by the APHA, while Southern City already embodied most of the policy recommendations. It was a matter of degree.

The second research question to which we sought an answer is, How would the public and community, state, and federal policy makers react to the idea of adopting these policies? We have documented that exceptionally strong support for most of the policies recommended by the APHA already exists among community, state, and federal respondents. Contraceptives and abortions without parental consent were the two policies receiving weakest support. The right to a first trimester abortion without parental consent has been established nationwide by the Supreme Court. The right to contraceptive care without requiring parental consent is being achieved on a state-by-state basis. The North Carolina legislature gave teenagers the right to contraceptive care in July 1977. Citizen attitudes, however, are lagging behind official support for making birth control services available to teenagers without parental consent.

Our third research question is, What are the points of view of the teenagers who are already using these services? The teenagers we interviewed affirmed the policies proposed by the APHA. We believe the teenagers' eight recommendations for change summarized in this chapter translate into affirmation of the need for and desirability of policies such as the APHA proposes.

Finally, we ask, If these APHA policies are adopted by communities, will they actually lead to successful community management of adolescent fertility rates? It is, of course, not possible to answer a definite yes on the basis of this study of two communities and one set of state and federal policy makers. A definite yes must await further studies in a variety of settings. In particular, the urban-rural dichotomies must be given extensive further study. We believe, however, that our study offers initial evidence that adoption of these APHA policies enables communities to manage adolescent fertility more successfully than communities that do not adopt these or equivalent policies.

The consistency with which Southern City was more successful than Farmville in lowering excess fertility among its sexually active teenagers seems to us to be convincing initial evidence that the policies studied here can effectively help communities reduce excess fertility rates among their sexually active teenagers.

APPENDIX A:
FIFTEEN STANDARDS FOR
AMBULATORY CARE OF
PREGNANT ADOLESCENTS

1. Adolescents are individuals and should be treated with respect and a nonjudgmental attitude, in an atmosphere of privacy and confidentiality.
2. Adolescents must be provided access to sex and family life education, contraceptive advice and treatment, and pregnancy testing, abortion, and prenatal/postpartum care without parental consent.
3. Adequate financial support should be available so that access to services is not restricted.
4. Provisions should be made for the early detection of pregnancy in adolescent women, and information concerning the availability of this service should be emphasized.
5. All alternatives for dealing with the pregnancy must be presented as viable solutions.
6. An interdisciplinary, comprehensive approach should be utilized in dealing with adolescent pregnancy.
7. Where appropriate and possible, services should be offered to the father of the child and to the adolescent's parents.
8. Early and consistent prenatal care should be available and accessible for those young women continuing their pregnancies to term.
9. The nutritional status of the adolescent should be assessed to ensure that appropriate counseling and services are provided.
10. Adequate preparation for the hospital and birth experience should be provided.
11. Postpregnancy care should be provided and should emphasize family planning services.
12. A program of consistent counseling and health education should be provided to the adolescent during and after the pregnancy.
13. The pregnant adolescent should be encouraged to continue her regular education and should be provided with the appropriate support services needed to do so.
14. Special classes in family life education should be provided for all adolescents, especially those pregnant adolescents who continue their pregnancy to term.
15. Programs for pregnant adolescents should undergo systematic, ongoing evaluation.

APPENDIX B:
INSTRUMENTS DEVELOPED FOR
THE STUDY

INSTRUMENT B:
STUDY OF ADOLESCENT PREGNANCIES

Instructions

In the first part of the questionnaire we have listed 20 ideas about things people in this county could do to help solve the problem of unmarried schoolgirls getting pregnant.

We are interested in learning your views on each of these ideas. First, in part a under each idea we want to find out how you personally feel about having each idea as a program or policy for your county. Second, in part b under each idea we want to find out how likely you believe it is that the people of your county would favor having the idea become a program or policy in your county.

For each of the stated ideas, circle first under Question a the number that best represents how strongly you favor or oppose the idea. Second, circle under Question b the number that best represents how likely you believe the people of your community would be to favor the idea.

1. Allowing information about sex only to persons over 18.

   a. How much do you personally favor or oppose this idea?

1	2	3	4	5
strongly favor	moderately favor	neither favor nor oppose; not sure	moderately oppose	strongly oppose

   b. How likely do you believe it is that the people of your community would favor this idea?

1	2	3	4	5
very likely	probably likely	neither likely nor unlikely; uncertain	probably unlikely	very unlikely

---

Instrument A is a shortened form of Instrument B.

243

2. Providing program funding so that the teenager can easily get contraception and abortion services.

    a. How much do you personally favor or oppose this idea?

1	2	3	4	5
strongly favor	moderately favor	neither favor nor oppose; not sure	moderately oppose	strongly oppose

    b. How likely do you believe it is that the people of your community would favor this idea?

1	2	3	5	5
very likely	probably likely	neither likely nor unlikely; uncertain	probably unlikely	very unlikely

3. Refusing abortions to anyone under 18.

    a. How much do you personally favor or oppose this idea?

1	2	3	4	5
strongly favor	moderately favor	neither favor nor oppose; not sure	moderately oppose	strongly oppose

    b. How likely do you believe it is that the people of your community would favor this idea?

1	2	3	4	5
very likely	probably likely	neither likely nor unlikely; uncertain	probably unlikely	very unlikely

4. Making contraceptive advice and services available to all teenagers.

    a. How much do you personally favor or oppose this idea?

1	2	3	4	5
strongly favor	moderately favor	neither favor nor oppose; not sure	moderately oppose	strongly oppose

    b. How likely do you believe it is that the people of your community would favor this idea?

1	2	3	4	5
very likely	probably likely	neither likely nor unlikely; uncertain	probably unlikely	very unlikely

5. Requesting pregnant girls to leave school before the fifth month of pregnancy.

   a. How much do you personally favor or oppose this idea?

1	2	3	4	5
strongly favor	moderately favor	neither favor nor oppose; not sure	moderately oppose	strongly oppose

   b. How likely do you believe it is that the people of your community would favor this idea?

1	2	3	4	5
very likely	probably likely	neither likely nor unlikely; uncertain	probably unlikely	very unlikely

6. Talking about all alternatives with the pregnant teenager (adoption, abortion, keeping child with marriage, keeping child without marriage).

   a. How much do you personally favor or oppose this idea?

1	2	3	4	5
strongly favor	moderately favor	neither favor nor oppose; not sure	moderately oppose	strongly oppose

   b. How likely do you believe it is that the people of your community would favor this idea?

1	2	3	4	5
very likely	probably likely	neither likely nor unlikely; uncertain	probably unlikely	very unlikely

7. Encouraging unmarried teenagers to accept responsibility for pregnancy by having the child.

   a. How much do you personally favor or oppose this idea?

1	2	3	4	5
strongly favor	moderately favor	neither favor nor oppose; not sure	moderately oppose	strongly oppose

   b. How likely do you believe it is that the people of your community would favor this idea?

1	2	3	4	5
very likely	probably likely	neither likely nor unlikely; uncertain	probably unlikely	very unlikely

8. Encouraging service programs to stress having teenage girls who believe they may be pregnant get a pregnancy test as early as possible.

a. How much do you personally favor or oppose this idea?

1	2	3	4	5
strongly favor	moderately favor	neither favor nor oppose; not sure	moderately oppose	strongly oppose

b. How likely do you believe it is that the people of your community would favor this idea?

1	2	3	4	5
very likely	probably likely	neither likely nor unlikely; uncertain	probably unlikely	very unlikely

9. Emphasize the teaching that sexual union outside of marriage is a sin.

1	2	3	4	5
strongly favor	moderately favor	neither favor nor oppose; not sure	moderately oppose	strongly oppose

b. How likely do you believe it is that the people of your community would favor this idea?

1	2	3	4	5
very likely	probably likely	neither likely nor unlikely; uncertain	probably unlikely	very unlikely

10. Providing teenagers contraceptive care without parental consent, if necessary.

a. How much do you personally favor or oppose this idea?

1	2	3	4	5
strongly favor	moderately favor	neither favor nor oppose; not sure	moderately oppose	strongly oppose

b. How likely do you believe it is that the people of your community would favor this idea?

1	2	3	4	5
very likely	probably likely	neither likely nor unlikely; uncertain	probably unlikely	very unlikely

11. Keeping sex education out of the schools.

   a. How much do you personally favor or oppose this idea?

1	2	3	4	5
strongly favor	moderately favor	neither favor nor oppose; not sure	moderately oppose	strongly oppose

   b. How likely do you believe it is that the people of your community would favor this idea?

1	2	3	4	5
very likely	probably likely	neither likely nor unlikely; uncertain	probably unlikely	very unlikely

12. Providing early and consistent visits to the doctor for teenage girls having a baby.

   a. How much do you personally favor or oppose this idea?

1	2	3	4	5
strongly favor	moderately favor	neither favor nor oppose; not sure	moderately oppose	strongly oppose

   b. How likely do you believe it is that the people of your community would favor this idea?

1	2	3	4	5
very likely	probably likely	neither likely nor unlikely; uncertain	probably unlikely	very unlikely

13. Making abortion available to teenagers.

   a. How much do you personally favor or oppose this idea?

1	2	3	4	5
strongly favor	moderately favor	neither favor nor oppose; not sure	moderately oppose	strongly oppose

   b. How likely do you believe it is that the people of your community would favor this idea?

1	2	3	4	5
very likely	probably likely	neither likely nor unlikely; uncertain	probably unlikely	very unlikely

14. Seeing to it that health, educational, nutritional, social service, and other providers work together to provide services to pregnant teenagers.

a. How much do you personally favor or oppose this idea?

1	2	3	4	5
strongly favor	moderately favor	neither favor nor oppose; not sure	moderately oppose	strongly oppose

b. How likely do you believe it is that the people of your community would favor this idea?

1	2	3	4	5
very likely	probably likely	neither likely nor unlikely; uncertain	probably unlikely	very unlikely

15. Restricting contraceptives to persons over 18.

a. How much do you personally favor or oppose this idea?

1	2	3	4	5
strongly favor	moderately favor	neither favor nor oppose; not sure	moderately oppose	strongly oppose

b. How likely do you believe it is that the people of your community would favor this idea?

1	2	3	4	5
very likely	probably likely	neither likely nor unlikely; uncertain	probably unlikely	very unlikely

16. Providing teenagers with sex education and family life education at school.

a. How much do you personally favor or oppose this idea?

1	2	3	4	5
strongly favor	moderately favor	neither favor nor oppose; not sure	moderately oppose	strongly oppose

b. How likely do you believe it is that the people of your community would favor this idea?

1	2	3	4	5
very likely	probably likely	neither likely nor unlikely; uncertain	probably unlikely	very unlikely

17. Allowing abortion for teenagers without parental consent, if necessary.

    a. How much do you personally favor or oppose this idea?

1	2	3	4	5
strongly favor	moderately favor	neither favor nor oppose; not sure	moderately oppose	strongly oppose

    b. How likely do you believe it is that the people of your community would favor this idea?

1	2	3	4	5
very likely	probably likely	neither likely nor unlikely; uncertain	probably unlikely	very unlikely

18. Keeping girls in their regular classes right up to childbirth and returning to school soon after the pregnancy has ended.

    a. How much do you personally favor or oppose this idea?

1	2	3	4	5
strongly favor	moderately favor	neither favor nor oppose; not sure	moderately oppose	strongly oppose

    b. How likely do you believe it is that the people of your community would favor this idea?

1	2	3	4	5
very likely	probably likely	neither likely nor unlikely; uncertain	probably unlikely	very unlikely

19. Encouraging courses about birth control for all students in junior high school.

    a. How much do you personally favor or oppose this idea?

1	2	3	4	5
strongly favor	moderately favor	neither favor nor oppose; not sure	moderately oppose	strongly oppose

    b. How likely do you believe it is that the people of your community would favor this idea?

1	2	3	4	5
very likely	probably likely	neither likely nor unlikely; uncertain	probably unlikely	very unlikely

20. Assigning responsibility for coordination of problem pregnancy services to one agency in the community.

    a. How much do you personally favor or oppose this idea?

1	2	3	4	5
strongly favor	moderately favor	neither favor nor oppose; not sure	moderately oppose	strongly oppose

    b. How likely do you believe it is that the people of your community would favor this idea?

1	2	3	4	5
very likely	probably likely	neither likely nor unlikely; uncertain	probably unlikely	very unlikely

We are interested in getting your impressions of what teenagers who are of junior high and high school age in your county do when they think they may be pregnant. What you do not know is as important for us to learn as what you do know about where school-age girls go for help, and we expect that very few persons will know answers for every question.

What Teenage Girls Do

1. Please give us your impression of what school-age girls in your county do when they suspect pregnancy (who they first talk to, where they go for help).

2. Please name places or persons to whom they turn for help.

    Place or Person   Service Provided

Pregnancy Tests

3. One of the first things a girl who thinks she may be pregnant can do is get a pregnancy test. Where do school-age girls who live in your county go to get pregnancy tests? (If you do not know these places, please write in "do not know"; if you think there is no place to get one, please write in "none available.")

Names of Places

a. _____

b. _____

c. _____

d. _____

Counseling

4. Some communities provide counseling to adolescents who become pregnant, in order to provide information and help them through the many decisions that confront them. What individuals or agencies either formally or informally provide counseling help to pregnant teenagers in your community? (If these services are available but you do not know who is providing them, please write in "do not know"; if you think none of these services are available, please write in "none available.")

Names of Individuals or Agencies

a. _____
b. _____
c. _____
d. _____
e. _____

Prenatal Care

5. If a teenager finds she is pregnant and decides to keep the baby, what services are available for her for prenatal care? (If you think there are services available but you do not know of them, please write in "do not know"; if you think there are no services available, please write in "none available.")

Name of Service   Description

a. _____   _____
b. _____   _____
c. _____   _____
d. _____   _____

Abortions

6. Sometimes pregnant teenagers choose to seek an abortion. Where do teenagers from your community who desire an abortion go to seek abortion services (either inside or outside the county)? (If these services are available but you do not know where they go to get them, please write in "do not know"; if you think these services are not available, please write in "none available.")

Names of Hospitals or Other Places

a. _____
b. _____
c. _____
d. _____

Contraceptive Services

7. What programs offer actual contraceptive services (birth control methods) to teenagers? (If you think there are programs that do this, but you do not know which ones, please write in "do not know"; if you think there are no programs that provide these services, please write in "none available.")

Names of Programs

a._____
b._____
c._____
d._____

Concerned Agencies

8. What agencies or groups in your community are working together or discussing ways of improving services to pregnant teenagers? (If some agencies or groups are doing these things, but you do not know which ones, please write in "do not know"; if you think none are doing these things, please write in "no one doing.")

Names of Agencies

a._____
b._____
c._____
d._____

9. What agencies or persons in the community would be interested in any expansion of community help to teenagers who become pregnant? (If you think some would be interested but you do not know exactly who, please write in "do not know"; if you think there is no one interested, please write in "none interested.")

Names of Persons of Agencies

a._____
b._____
c._____
d._____

Difficulties Encountered

10. What difficulties, if any, do pregnant teenagers in your county most often experience in obtaining abortion or prenatal services? (If you do not know of any difficulties being had, please write in "do not know.")

1. Abortion Services (please list difficulties)

a. _____
b. _____
c. _____
d. _____

2. Prenatal Services (please list difficulties)

a. _____
b. _____
c. _____
d. _____

Recommendations for Changes

11. If you think additional resources, changes, laws, or policies are needed in your county to better serve the pregnant adolescent, would you name the two or three most important? (If you do not think any of these are needed, please write in "none needed.")

Needed Resources, Changes, Laws, Policies

a. _____
b. _____
c. _____
d. _____

Left-Out Information

12. We hope to be able to piece together a picture of where teenagers who are or think they may be pregnant go for help and to find out what services are available to them. What other pieces of information or ideas do you feel may help us achieve this? (If you cannot think of anything else, please write in "do not know.")

Further Information or Ideas

a. _____
b. _____
c. _____

Others to Interview

13. We plan to interview several persons in your county who know a lot about or who are concerned about pregnancies among school-girls. Who do you think are the two or three most important persons or agencies we should try to interview? (If you cannot think of any, please write in "none known.")

Names of Persons or Agencies

a. _____

b. _____

c. _____

d. _____

PERSONAL DATA

Please answer the following 12 questions. This information is strictly confidential. It will be used only to make group comparisons.

1. What is the year of your birth? _____ (please write the year in the blank)

2. What is your sex? Female   Male (please circle your answer)

3. Have you ever been married? Yes   No (please circle your answer)

   a. If yes, please give the date of your marriage (if married more than once, the date of your first marriage)_____
   b. If yes, are you currently divorced or separated? Yes   No (please circle your answer)

4. Do you have any children?   Yes No (please circle your answer)

   a. If yes, how many? _____ (please put number in blank)
   b. If yes, please list their ages: Boys' ages: ,   ,   ,
      Girls' ages: ,   ,   ,

5. If you have no children, are you or your spouse expecting? Yes   No (please circle your answer

6. Of what church are you a member?_____
   (please write in church name; if none, please write "none")

7. How much school have you completed to the present? (please circle the highest year completed)

   | Grammar School | High School |
   | 1 2 3 4 5 6 7 8 9 | 10   11   12 |

   | College | Graduate School |
   | 13   14   15   16 | 17   18   19   20   21   22 |

8. Other than the formal schooling in question 7, have you had other training or educational experience? (for example, technical or business school)

   Yes   No (please circle your answer)
   If yes, please list what type of training and where you were trained:

9. What is your race? (please circle your answer)
   Black   White   Other

10. Please name your occupation or job title:

    a. _____(please write this in the blank)
    b. If not working, please write in whether you are a housewife,
       retired, disabled, or temporarily unemployed, using the
       blank above.

11. What was your total family income before taxes in 1976? (Include
    all sources of income for all family household members.) (please
    check the space beside your answer)

    a._____under $5,000
    b._____between $5,000 and $10,000
    c._____between $10,000 and $15,000
    d._____between $15,000 and $25,000
    e._____over $25,000

INSTRUMENT C:
MEDICAL SERVICE PROVIDERS

1. In what setting(s) do you provide contraceptive information and
   advice for adolescent women under 18? Check as many as apply.

   Private practice office
   Family planning clinics   _____
   Teen clinics   _____
   Schools   _____
   Other (please specify)_____
   None provided   _____

2. Do you offer contraceptive services (such as pills, IUDs) to teenagers?

   Yes   _____
   No   _____
   Other (please specify)_____

3. Do you offer problem pregnancy counseling (advice on and referrals for adoption, abortion, financial assistance, other matters)?

   Yes   _____
   No   _____
   Other (please specify)_____
   Do not know   _____

4. Do you do pregnancy testing for teenagers?

Yes _____
No _____
Other (please specify)_____
Do not know _____

5. Regarding parental consent, please check the columns that apply to your services to teenagers.

Service	Require Parental Consent	Do not Require if Emancipated Teen	Parental Consent Unnecessary
Counseling			
Contraception			
Pregnancy testing			
First trimester abortion			
Prenatal services			
Other			

6. Do you offer prenatal services to pregnant teenagers?

Yes _____
No _____
Other (please specify)_____
Do not know _____

7. If you offer prenatal services, do you have a separate prenatal clinic for teenagers?

Yes _____
No _____
Other (please specify)_____
Do not know _____

8. Do you offer education in nutrition for pregnant teenagers?

Yes _____
No _____
Other (please specify)_____
Do not know _____

9. If you offer prenatal services to teenagers, is any attention given to preparing them for the hospital experience?

Yes _____
No _____
Do not offer prenatal care _____
Other (please specify)_____

10. If you offer postpregnancy care or checkups, do you emphasize family planning services?

    Yes   _____

    No   _____

    Do not offer postpregnancy care   _____

    Other (please specify)_____

11. In your estimation, what percent of teenagers in this county who have problem pregnancies and who might want an abortion are prevented from getting one because of the lack of money?

12. What difficulties, other than lack of money, do you encounter in assisting your clients in obtaining abortions, if that is what they choose?

13. In your estimation, what percent of pregnant teenagers are unable to obtain proper prenatal care in your county because of a lack of money?

14. What difficulties, other than lack of money, do you encounter in assisting your clients in obtaining prenatal care, if they choose to carry the pregnancy to term?

INSTRUMENT E
COUNSELORS' FORM

1. Do you require parental consent for counseling and referral services to people under 18? (check as many as apply)

   Parental consent required   _____

   Parental consent not required   _____

   No parental consent required if teenager is
     emancipated   _____

   Other (please specify)_____

   Do not know   _____

2. If you counsel teenagers, which of the following alternatives to a problem pregnancy do you explain? (check as many as apply)

   Adoption   _____

   Abortion   _____

   Keeping child with marriage   _____

   Keeping child without marriage   _____

   Do not counsel in this area   _____

   Other (please specify)_____

Ministers' form, Instrument D, is similar.

3. If you counsel pregnant teenagers, of the pregnant teenagers (under 18) you have counseled during the past 12 months, please estimate the percent of decisions made in these four categories.

Adoption _____
Abortion _____
Keeping child with marriage _____
Keeping child without marriage _____
Cannot estimate _____

4. Do you involve the parents of the girls or the fathers of the children in your work with pregnant teenagers?

Yes, both _____
Parents only _____
Father of child _____
No _____

5. Please list the sources of money that are available in your county to assist teenagers in paying for an abortion.

Sources of Financial Help

a._____
b._____
c._____
d._____
No financial help is available _____
Do not know _____

6. In your estimation, what percent of teenagers with problem pregnancies in your county who want an abortion are prevented from getting one because of lack of money?

Estimated percent _____
Do not know _____

7. What difficulties, other than lack of money, do you encounter in assisting your clients in obtaining an abortion, if that is what they choose?

8. Please estimate the percent of pregnant teenagers in your county who were able unable to obtain prenatal care because of lack of money during the past 12 months.

Estimated percent _____
Do not know _____

9. What difficulties, other than lack of money, do you encounter in assisting your clients in obtaining prenatal care, if they choose to carry the pregnancy to term?

10. How have teenagers you have counseled regarding a problem pregnancy learned of your service?

Yourself _____

Public information announcements _____

Minister _____

School personnel _____

Acquaintance of the teenager _____

Parent of the teenager _____

Other (please specify)_____

Unknown _____

11. Please estimate the number of teenagers with problem pregnancies whom you have counseled within the past 12 months?

12. To what clinics, hospitals, doctors, or services do you refer teenagers who select the option of abortion?

a._____

b._____

c._____

d._____

e._____

Do not refer teenagers for abortions _____

Other (please specify)_____

Do not know _____

13. To what clinics, hospitals, doctors, or services do you refer teenagers who decide to have the baby for prenatal care?

Name of Individual, Service, or Institution

a._____

b._____

c._____

d._____

e._____

Do not refer teenagers for above services _____

Other (please specify)_____

INSTRUMENT F:
PHARMACISTS' INTERVIEW SCHEDULE

1. What role do you play as a pharmacist in providing contraceptives and family planning advice to junior high- and high school-age persons through your pharmacy?

2. In what ways do you assist junior high- and high school-age persons who are seeking birth control information and contraceptives?

   a. Information assistance

   b. Provision of contraceptives

   c. Other roles or assistance

3. Can you estimate the number of junior high- and high school-age persons who purchase contraceptives through your drugstore?

   _____
   (number)

4. Generally are more contraceptives (of all kinds) being purchased, and particularly, are more being purchased by younger persons? _____ Please describe any trends you see in the volume of purchases and the age of purchasers.

5. Please estimate the volume of contraceptives sold in the county in each of the past five years and the percentage of each yearly volume you would attribute to junior high school- and high school-age purchasers.

	Volume of Contraceptive Purchases					
Year	Pills	IUD	Diaphragm	Condom	Foam, Jelly, or Cream	Other
1972						
1973						
1974						
1975						
1976						

6. Please describe how you see the roles of the pharmacists, physicians, hospitals, and any other providers in meeting the birth control needs of junior high- and high school-age persons who are sexually active.

INSTRUMENT G:
SCHOOL STUDY

1. Does your school offer sex education to the students?

   Yes (go to question 1a) _____
   No (go to question 2) _____

1a. What percent of the students in your school receive sex education?

   Percent _____
   Do not know _____

1b. At what grade level(s) is this instruction offered?

1c. In what course(s) is sex education offered?

   Course name(s)

   Other (please specify)_____

   (go to question 3)

2. Is sex education prohibited by policy in your school?

   Yes _____
   No _____

3. Do you have a program especially designed for pregnant girls in your school?

   Yes (go to question 3a) _____
   No (go to question 4) _____

3a. What is the goal of your program for pregnant girls?

3b. Are social work services provided for the girls in the program by a school social worker or a social worker brought in by the school from another agency?

   Yes _____
   No _____
   Other (please specify)_____

3c. Are any other agencies, such as the social services or Health Department, directly involved in the program?

   Yes (please specify)_____
   No _____

3d. Is a pregnant schoolgirl allowed to choose to attend under the regular curriculum rather than a special program?

   Yes _____
   No _____
   Only under special circumstances (please specify)_____

3e. What has been the range in the size of enrollment in the program during the past year?

3f. Is transportation to school provided for all those eligible for the program?

Yes _____

No _____

Other (please specify)_____

3g. Is nutrition education a part of the program?

Yes _____

No _____

Other (please specify)_____

3h. Is family life education (home economics, parenting, marriage expectations) a part of the program?

Yes _____

No _____

Other (please specify)_____

3i. Is education in the use of contraceptives and family planning a part of the program?

Yes _____

No _____

Other (please specify)_____

3j. What additional resources (people, money, other), if any, does your program need to reach its goal more fully? (go to question 5)

4. For those schools that do not have a program especially designed for pregnant girls, please list any special considerations that are given to pregnant girls (flexible attendance hours, social work services, counseling, other).

5. What educational alternatives are open to pregnant girls in your school? (check all that apply)

Continue in regular classes until they stop of their
  own accord _____

Continue in regular classes until they are asked to
  stop by the school _____

Quit school, even if under 16, without official pressure to return _____

Enter special program for pregnant girls _____

Other (please specify)_____

6. Are students who are mothers given any special consideration in the school? (check all that apply)

No _____
Flexible attendance hours _____
Social work services _____
Special classes _____
Other (please specify)_____

7. In regard to sex education, does your school (system) have a policy (either written or unwritten) on sex education in the curriculum?

Yes (go to question 7a) _____
No (go to question 8) _____

7a. Is your policy a written policy?

Yes (if possible, please send us a copy) _____
No _____

7b. Who made your policy on sex education in the curriculum?

8. Who in your school might be likely to talk with girls about a problem pregnancy, either formally or informally?

INSTRUMENT H:
PERSONAL RESPONSE QUESTION SET

1. When someone asked you your reaction to being pregnant, the word that best describes how you felt is:

upset _____ angry _____
relaxed _____ proud _____
embarrassed _____ other _____
_____ (write in)_____

2. Who was the first person you talked to about your pregnancy?

I did not talk to anyone _____ my boyfriend _____
my mother _____ another friend _____
my father _____ other _____
_____ (write in)_____

3. Other people I talked with about my pregnancy were: (check as many as appropriate)

no one else _____ my minister, priest, or rabbi _____
my husband _____ a family planning worker _____
my boyfriend _____ a social worker _____
my father _____ a guidance counselor _____
my mother _____ other persons _____
_____ (write in)_____

4. At first, I was very careful not to let the following persons know of my pregnancy: (check as many as appropriate)

    everyone ____   my minister, priest, or rabbi ____
    my husband ____   a family planning worker ____
    my boyfriend ____   a social worker ____
    my father ____   a guidance counselor ____
    my mother ____   other persons ____
                           (write in)_____

5. How did each of the following people feel about your decision to have your baby?

    your sexual partner: I did not have a boyfriend ____
                          He did not know about the pregnancy ____
                          He preferred that I have the baby ____
                          He did not care what I did ____
                          He preferred that I have an abortion ____
                          Other ____
                          (write in)_____

    your mother: She did not know about the pregnancy ____
                          She preferred that I have the baby ____
                          She did not care what I did ____
                          She preferred that I have an abortion ____
                          Other ____
                          (write in)_____

    your father: He did not know about the pregnancy ____
                          He preferred that I have the baby ____
                          He did not care what I did ____
                          He preferred that I have an abortion ____
                          Other ____
                          (write in)_____

6. When I became pregnant, the contraceptive method I was using was:

    none ____   condoms (rubbers) ____
    pills ____   rhythm (counting days) ____
    diaphragm ____   withdrawal (pulling out) ____
    foam, jelly, or cream ____   other ____
                                 (write in)_____

7. I was using that contraceptive method:

    all the time _____
    sometimes _____
    not at all _____

8. When I got pregnant:

I wanted to get pregnant   _____
I did not care if I got pregnant   _____
I did not want to get pregnant   _____

9. I _____ using contraceptives (choose one answer):

like (using contraceptives)
do not like (using contraceptives)
do not care about (using contraceptives)

10. How did the man by whom you were pregnant feel about using contraceptives?

I do not know how he felt   _____
He was in favor of using contraceptives   _____
He was not in favor of using contraceptives   _____
He did not care one way or the other   _____
Other   _____
(write in)_____

11. My present relationship with the man who got me pregnant is:

We are no longer talking to each other   _____
We are still talking to each other, but less than before_____
Our relationship is the same as before   _____
We are closer now than before   _____

12. Including this last pregnancy, I have been pregnant:

only once   _____
two times   _____
three times   _____
more than three times   _____

13. I found out I was pregnant:

less than a week after I missed my first period   _____
1-3 weeks after I missed my first period   _____
about 1 month after I missed my first period   _____
about 3 months after I missed my first period _____

14. I went for a pregnancy test:

immediately after I suspected I was pregnant   _____
one to two months after I suspected I was pregnant _____
I never had a pregnancy test   _____

15. If you had a pregnancy test, where did you have it done?

public health clinic _____

a hospital _____

a private doctor _____

I did not have a pregnancy test _____

16. The man by whom I was pregnant was:

my husband

my boyfriend _____

someone else _____

_____

17. I began prenatal care in the:

first or second month	____	seventh month	____
third month	____	eighth month	____
fourth month	____	I had no prenatal care	____
fifth month	____	Other	____
sixth month	____	(write in)_____	

18. I made about _____ prenatal visits:

one	____	11 to 13	____
two to four	____	14 to 16	____
five to seven	____	more than 16	____
eight to ten	____	I made no prenatal visits	____

19. I am _____ years old:

11		15	
12	____	16	____
13	____	17	____
14	____	18	____
	____	other	____

20. I am now:

single	____	living together (not legally married)	
married	____		
divorced	____	widowed	____
separated	____	other (write in)_____	____

21. My present occupation is:

working full-time	____	in school	____
working part-time	____	keeping house	____
unemployed	____	other	____
		(write in)_____	

22. The highest grade I have finished in school is:

eighth grade	____	eleventh grade	____
ninth grade	____	twelfth grade	____
tenth grade	____	some college	____

23. I am presently living with:

my husband	____	my father	____
my boyfriend	____	both parents	____
another relative	____	alone	____
my roommate	____	other	____
my mother	____	(write in)_____	

24. I have lived in Farmville for:

less than one year	____	more than three years but	
one to two years	____	not always	____
two to three years	____	all of my life	____

INSTRUMENT I:
HEURISTIC ELICITATION QUESTION FRAME

1. How did you first suspect you were pregnant? Who was the first person to suspect your pregnancy?

2. What alternatives did you consider? Any others? (Probe for consideration of action: pregnancy test, abortion, marriage, prenatal care, do nothing.)

3. Who did you first tell about your pregnancy? Who else? Anyone else?

4. What advice did _____ give you? What else did _____ tell you?

5. When did you tell _____ about your pregnancy?

6. What places or persons did _____ recommend where you could go for help? Any others?

7. What places did you know about where you could go for help?

8. Besides these places, what other people in the community might you ask for help in taking care of you and your baby during your pregnancy?

9. To what places or persons did you finally go for help?

10. Would you describe for me the kind of care or help given to you at _____ (name of place) or by _____ (name of person)?

11. What were your reasons for deciding to keep your baby rather than having it adopted?

12. What were your reasons for deciding to keep your baby rather than having it aborted?

13. Who does the baby stay with most of the time? Who else takes care of the baby? Who else? When?

14. What other girls around your age do you know about who have been pregnant recently?

15. What did _____ (name of girl) do about the pregnancy?

16. If you were asked to help design a program to meet the needs of teenagers in the areas of family planning, pregnancy, and child care, what things would you suggest? (Probes: classes—what type, what should be taught, should they include girls and guys, would the guys come? Do you think it should be for all teenagers, or just for some? Which ones? Where should such a program be held, who should sponsor it?)

APPENDIX C:
DETAILED DESCRIPTION OF
RESULTS OBTAINED AND
METHODOLOGY

PRETEST

The testing procedure planned for the two communities was pre-tested in two similar communities of comparable size and rural-urban characteristics within the 11-county health systems area. The primary instruments for the research were the 20 questions focused on the American Public Health Association (APHA) standards and 13 questions probing what respondents believed to be the network of care within each study community. These instruments were mailed to a sample of 75 respondents chosen on the basis planned for Farmville and Southern City. The response rates and answers to individual items in the instruments were used to establish the overall sample size plans for the two local community studies and to revise the wording of several questions that had unclear response patterns in the pretest sample.

INTERVIEW PROCEDURES

Personal interviews constituted the basic and most important community study technique used in this research. The strengths and weaknesses of the study lie mainly in the soundness of the theoretical specification of the study populations and the conduct of the interviews. The decisions about whom to interview were important methodologically in the research. Basically, we sought to interview every person in the rural community who, we believed, had any relevant part in the community effort to manage adolescent fertility. Having made that decision, we defined the study population by our perceptions of who those persons might be. This resulted in our decision to interview the numerous policy makers, service providers, and teenagers described below. Other persons and groups were interviewed as they became known to the researchers during the study.

Our policy was to interview all members of any board or governmental body seen to be related to adolescent fertility behaviors in the community. The interview policy for staff members of agencies was to interview as many or as few as were believed by the staff of each agency to have anything to do with adolescent fertility. For example, in Farmville we interviewed the total staff of seven social workers in the Department of Social Services because every member of the

staff handled cases involving adolescent fertility control, for contraceptive assistance, sex education, or abortion, if needed. In contrast, only two members of the Department of Mental Health were
seen by their agency head and staff members with whom we talked as
having any activities relevant to adolescent fertility. Similarly, a
significant number of the staff members of the public school administration were interviewed because 11 staff members were viewed as
having activities relevant to adolescent fertility. At times it was
necessary to be arbitrary in limiting the number of interviews to a
manageable size. For example, we decided to interview all local
school principals in Farmville, but to interview only the four school
counselors viewed by the school administrators as the most active in
the area of helping adolescents manage their fertility.

Thus it was a matter of judgment as to how many persons to interview in each category. Our research goal was to interview as many
persons as feasible in each category who, we believed, were important to the communities' efforts to manage adolescent fertility. There
were, for example, more than 40 medical doctors in Farmville. We
interviewed the 7 or the 13 gynecologists and family practice physicians who were the most involved in providing contraceptive services
and performing abortions. It was neither feasible nor desirable, from
our point of view, to interview every physician in the community.
Orthopedists and radiologists have no immediate relationship to the
network of community care for managing adolescent fertility. Our
goal in every case was to interview as many persons in every open-
ended category, such as physicians and school counselors, as we concluded were necessary to obtain a full view of what was happening in
that community. For closed categories, such as the human services
boards, county commissioners, or the school board, we interviewed
every member who would permit an interview or who was not on vacation.

While it was possible to interview a very high percentage of persons seen as having relevance to the community's efforts to manage
fertility among teenagers in Farmville, it was not possible to interview on such a broad basis in Southern City, where there were many
more members on each board and many more persons potentially in-
terviewable in each category. Our policy in Southern City was to interview as many persons on each board or in each category as had
been interviewed in Farmville. The persons picked for interview
were judged by the agency head or board chairman as being the most
informed or concerned about adolescent pregnancy.

RANDOM SAMPLING PROCEDURES

Random sampling was used to obtain responses from the general
public in the two communities. Our goal was to produce a sample of

TABLE C.1

Results of General Public Samples in Farmville and Southern City, 1977

	Farmville	Southern City
Original names drawn	750	750
Bad addresses		
Introductory letter returned	52	95
Undeliverable questionnaires	116	125
Returned blank	15	14
Refused	0	2
Never responded	333	299
Returned usable questionnaires	234	215
Response rate (percent)	40	40
Teenage respondents		
Questionnaires mailed	95	61
Responses	10	13
Nonresponses	85	48
Response rate (percent)	11	21
(combined response rate 15 percent)		

Source: Compiled by the author.

the general public that would include a completed response of 200 usable questionnaires. In order to accomplish this, we began by selecting 750 names (based on the return rates in the pretest), using random number tables for each of the two communities. The most recent county directory and city directory listed every male and female aged 18 and over living in the two communities. Each person was given an equal chance of being selected for the study.

These original 750 persons selected in each community resulted in the desired minimum number of respondents, as Table C.1 shows. In all, 234 usable responses were received from Farmville and 215 from Southern City. The response rate in each case was 40 percent. Questionnaires were mailed to parents who indicated that they had teenage children, one questionnaire for each teenager. The response to 95 questionnaires mailed to Farmville teenagers was a disappointing

10 (or 11 percent), while the response to the 61 questionnaires mailed to Southern City was a slightly more encouraging 13 (or 21 percent). Since questionnaires were sent to the parents of the teenagers with a letter asking them to pass the questionnaires on to their teenage children, it is impossible to know what percentage of the questionnaires were actually placed into the hands of the teenagers. We felt it was inappropriate to mail directly to the teenagers, since we had indicated full anonymity to the parents who responded, thus leaving it to them to decide whether to permit their teenagers to consider participating in the study.

The senior author conducted the interviewing in Farmville, and interviewing in Southern City was done primarily by trained interviewers. We made approximately five attempts to contact each person for an interview before declaring the individual unavailable. The junior author conducted all interviews and 15 reinterviews with teenage Farmville women who delivered in 1976.

Follow-up efforts with the mailed questionnaires to the general public and to the state and national policy makers and human services administrators consisted of a letter approximately two weeks after the first copy of the questionnaire was mailed. We sent respondents a second copy of the questionnaire in the follow-up letter.

We now turn to a detailed discussion of the results of interviewing efforts in the two local communities and the mailed questionnaires to the general public, state, and national study populations.

INTERVIEW AND MAILED QUESTIONNAIRE RESULTS

The tables below give the actual number of respondents in each category within the study and the percentage of success these numbers represent in terms of the number of interviews or mailed responses we sought. Whether we sought to interview all the persons in any one group or to get responses from a positionally defined subgroup is indicated in each case throughout the discussion of the interviewing and mailed questionnaire efforts.

Individual Teenagers

A major goal of our research was to be able to compare the experiences that adolescents actually had in the care network of the two communities with the care network that community policy makers and service providers believed existed. The best way to achieve this comparison was to specify a study population known to have needed or used the service system. We arbitrarily chose to interview all younger

TABLE C.2

Details of Study Population with Percentage of Responses on
Attitudes and Beliefs Related to APHA Standards for Management of
Adolescent Pregnancies, Farmville and Southern City, 1977

	Farmville		Southern City	
	Number	Percent Inter- viewed[a]	Number	Percent Inter- viewed[a]
Policy makers				
County commissioners	4	80		
City council	8	100		
Health board	1	50	6	100
Social services board	3	71	3	100
Mental health board	8	100	8	100
School board	7	88	9	100
School administrators	11	100	10	100
Ministerial Association	12	100	5	35
Other ministers	8	100		
Named influentials	10	100	3	50
Service providers				
Medical doctors	7		8	27
Other medical profes- sionals	1			
Health Department staff	6	100	8	100
Social services staff	9	100	6	100
Mental health staff	2	100	3	100
Pharmacists	7	100	5	100
School counselors	4	—[b]	3	—[b]

[a]Denotes percent obtained of number of interviews or mailed
questionnaires desired.
[b]Total number unknown.

Source: Compiled by the author.

teenagers in the two communities who gave birth during the calendar year 1976. We chose 1976 because it was the latest year for which data were available when the study began. In addition, interviews provided responses from that group of individuals who had most recently encountered the service system as recipients or potential recipients.

In addition to the teenagers mentioned above, we sought to obtain a sample of teenagers through the random selection from among all the teenagers in the two communities. Through these procedures we were able to obtain interviews with teenage mothers in each of the two communities plus teenage respondents from the general public. The response rate from the teenage general public was disappointing. As mentioned above, it is impossible to tell whether the teenagers themselves declined to participate in the study or whether their parents did not give them the questionnaires.

We feel that the sample of teenagers who gave birth in 1976 is very usable. On the other hand, the teenagers who responded as part of the general public provided only anecdotal information.

General Public

Table C.3 gives demographic data on the general public samples obtained in the two communities. Table C.4 provides comparisons between the demographic makeup of the actual population and the general public respondents in our sample. These comparisons will enable the reader to take the differences into account when studying the data. Comparative data are available on age, race, and sex.

As Table C.4 shows, in Farmville there was underrepresentation of persons in their twenties and of persons 60 and over. Persons in their forties were overrepresented by 9.3 percent, which may reflect a stronger interest in the subject of pregnancies among adolescents, since these persons are most likely to be parents of adolescents. In Southern City there were only minor variations between our sample population and the actual population, the greatest being an underrepresentation of persons in their twenties. On balance, the returned questionnaires seemed to match the actual profile of the general population within functional limits. Blacks were underrepresented in the Farmville responses by 18.9 percent, and by 17 percent in the responses from Southern City. Males were underrepresented by 11.5 percent in the Farmville returned sample and by 14 percent in Southern City. A higher rate of illiteracy for blacks, especially in Farmville, may have accounted in part for the lower response from blacks in both study groups. We believe that the data from the two communities are analyzed along enough dimensions in

TABLE C.3

Demographic Profile of General Public Respondents in Farmville and Southern City, 1977

	Farmville		Southern City	
	Number (N = 334)	Percent	Number (N = 215)	Percent
Race				
White	207	87	180	84
Black	19	8	23	11
Unknown	11	3	15	5
Sex				
Male	76	32	73	34
Female	151	64	137	64
Unknown	10	4	5	2
Education				
Less than high school	57	24	29	13
High school graduate	71	30	60	28
College	98	41	87	41
Graduate school	11	5	39	18
Religion				
Conservative Protestant	28	12	26	12
Mainline Protestant	155	66	117	54
Roman Catholic	7	3	11	5
Jewish	0	0	1	1
Other	35	15	49	23
Unknown	12	4	11	5
Age				
20 to 29	47	20	48	22
30 to 39	44	19	53	25
40 to 49	59	25	34	16
50 to 59	51	21	39	18
60 and over	24	10	31	14
Unknown	17	5	10	5
Number of children				
None	47	20	60	28
1 or 2	114	48	96	45
3 or more	76	32	59	27
Pregnancy status at marriage				
Pregnant	16	7	19	9
Not pregnant	155	65	135	63
Unknown	66	28	61	28
Occupation				
Professional	36	15	45	21
Manager	56	24	42	19
Clerical	34	14	28	13
Service	19	8	23	11
Blue collar	33	14	9	4
Unemployed	57	24	68	32
Other	2	1		
Aged children 11 to 19				
Yes	62	26	n.a.	
No	163	69	n.a.	
Unknown	12	5	n.a.	
Income				
Under $5,000	n.a.		14	7
$5,000-9,999	n.a.		27	12
$10,000-14,999	n.a.		38	18
$15,000-24,999	n.a.		64	30
$25,000 and over	n.a.		52	24
Unknown	n.a.		20	9

n.a. = not available

Source: Compiled by the author.

TABLE C.4

Percentage Differences between Actual Populations of Farmville and Southern City and the Percent of General Public Respondents, by Age, Race, and Sex, 1976

Age	Actual Population Number	Actual Population Percent	Percent Population Sampled	Percent Difference
Farmville, July 1, 1976				
20 to 29	5,448	25.0	21.4	−3.6
30 to 39	4,269	19.7	20.0	+0.3
40 to 49	3,794	17.5	26.8	+9.3
50 to 59	3,597	16.6	23.1	+6.5
60 and over	4,546	20.9	10.9	−10.0
Total aged 20 and over	21,654			
Southern City, July 1, 1976				
20 to 29	55,578	32.0	23.4	−8.6
30 to 39	37,125	21.4	25.8	+4.4
40 to 49	28,682	16.5	16.7	+0.2
50 to 59	24,042	13.8	19.0	+5.2
60 and over	27,998	16.1	15.1	−1.0
Total aged 20 and over	173,401			
Differences by Race and Sex				
Farmville blacks	—	28.0	9.1	−18.9
Southern City blacks	—	29.7	12.7	−17.0
Farmville males	15,781	47.5	36.0	−11.5
Farmville females	17,402	52.5	64.0	+11.5
Southern City males	132,315	49.0	35.0	−14.0
Southern City females	137,199	51.0	65.0	+14.0

Source: Compiled by the author.

later chapters to allow for reasonable understanding of the biases introduced by the observed differences between the estimated actual population and the sample population. We chose not to weight our sample results based on the July 1976 population estimates because the population estimates were themselves based on projection from the 1970 census and had a degree of error for which it was impossible to compensate accurately.

State of North Carolina

The persons and groups studied at the state level represented equivalents of persons and groups interviewed at the local level, except for the addition of judges. Judges were added because they have had significant influence on the availability of sex education, contraceptives, and abortions to teenagers in the United States. Response rates varied between 61 percent for the district court judges and 86 percent for the state supreme court judges. The overall response rate for judges was 62 percent, weighted heavily by the large number of district court judges in the sample who were nonrespondents. All North Carolina state legislators were included in the study: 54 percent of the state senators and 62 percent of the state representatives responded. Among human services administrators a gratifying 100 percent returned the questionnaires. Two of these were incomplete, however, and were not used in the final calculations. (See Table C.5.)

When compared with typical response rates achieved for studies of legislators conducted at such places as the Institute for Research in Social Sciences at the University of North Carolina at Chapel Hill, our obtained response rate was considered as good as can normally be achieved short of aggressively seeking interviews with each legislator. The total response from the governor's office and the 56 human services administrators represented all the top administrative decision makers in the state human services offices that we believed had impacts on the efforts of communities to manage adolescent fertility levels.

Federal Level

Responses from the federal executive and legislative branches were disappointing. Most congressmen wrote letters indicating that they adhered to a firm policy of not responding to any questionnaires that came to their offices, no matter what the subject matter or who the sponsor. The responses from 11 senators and 72 congressmen could not be used as representative of the entire Congress, but they

TABLE C.5

Details of Study Population with Percentage of Responses on
Attitudes and Beliefs Related to APHA Standards for Management of
Adolescent Pregnancies, State of North Carolina, 1977

	Number Returned	Percent Returned
Judges		
State supreme court	6	86
Circuit court of appeals	6	67
Superior court	29	64
District court	74	61
Congress		
State senators	27	54
State representatives	74	62
Human services administrators		
Governor, lieutenant governor	2	100
Department of Human Resources, top administrators	4	100
Administrative heads		
State Health Department	15	100
Department of Social Services	8	100
Department of Mental Health	11	100*
Department of Youth Services	3	100
Department of Public Instruction	11	100
Regional offices, administrative heads	4	100

*Includes two incomplete questionnaires returned and not used.

Source: Compiled by the author.

TABLE C.6

Details of Study Population with Percentage of Responses on
Attitudes and Beliefs Related to APHA Standards for Management of
Adolescent Pregnancies, Federal Level, 1977

	Number Returned	Percent Returned
Executive branch		
President and cabinet	0	0
White House office staff	2	29
Congress		
Senators	11	11
Representatives	72	17
Human services administrators		
Office of the Secretary (HEW)	2	50
Office of Assistant Secretary for Human Development	1	25
Office of Assistant Secretary for Legislation	4	80
Office of Assistant Secretary for Planning and Evaluation	3	75
Office of Assistant Secretary for Education	3	100
Office of Education	1	25
Office of Assistant Secretary for Health	2	100
Alcohol, Drug Abuse, and Mental Health Administration	3	75
Center for Disease Control	12	100
Food and Drug Administration	1	100
Health Resources Administration	3	60
Health Services Administration	4	100
National Institutes of Health	2	50
Health Care Finance Administration	1	100
Social Security Administration	2	100
Office of Child Support Enforcement	1	100
HEW regional directors	8	80
Overall response rate		76

Source: Compiled by the author.

did provide some interesting comparisons with state legislator attitudes and beliefs on the subjects in the questionnaire. (See Table
C.6.)

As on the state level, the federal human services administrators' response rate was gratifying. The top administrators in each
of the federal offices already studied at the local and state levels responded at an overall rate of 76 percent. It was especially gratifying
that eight of the ten regional directors of the Department of Health,
Education and Welfare replied.

APPENDIX D:
RADICAL DIFFERENCES IN
FEMALE ADOLESCENT ATTITUDES TOWARD
PREGNANCY AND
ITS IMMEDIATE CONSEQUENCES

Im summarizing attitudes toward pregnancy and its immediate consequences among teens who choose to have their babies instead of having an abortion, there are certain characteristics that break along racial lines. These characteristics were apparent to us despite all of our attempts to treat the problem of early pregnancy as an adolescent rather than a racial problem. What is interesting is the nature of the characteristic. The principal differences were in how white and black teenagers handled education and marriage. The interviews with teenagers suggested that there were thoughtful reasons behind the behaviors of both blacks and whites.

In the research sample for both Farmville and Southern City there was a marked tendency for black teenagers to have completed more education than their white counterparts (Table D. 1). The average years of school completed by 18-year-olds in Farmville was 10.7 years for whites and 11.3 years for blacks. In Southern City the differences were less pronounced. Black 18-year-olds had completed 11.4 years of school, compared with 11.1 years for white 18-year-olds. What the data and interviews with teenagers suggested was that

TABLE D. 1

Average Number of School Years Completed by Black and White
Teenage Mothers, Southern City and Farmville, 1976

Age	Southern City		Farmville	
	Black	White	Black	White
18	11.40	11.1	11.3	10.70
17	10.25	10.3	11.8	10.25
16	9.60	9.3	9.7	10.00
15	9.10	9.0	9.0	9.00
14	7.70	—	7.5	—
13	8.00	—	—	—

Source: Compiled by the author.

black teenagers continued their schooling even after interrupting it for pregnancy and childbearing. White girls who delivered in their teens seemed less apt to return to school.

Beverly Coors told the interviewer that her greatest concern during her pregnancy was how she would finish school. She was the youngest of four daughters. The others had gotten their high school diplomas; and Mrs. Coors was determined that Beverly would be able to complete high school, too. She agreed to help out with the new baby so that her daughter could finish. At the time of one of the interviews, Beverly had just graduated, and she and her mother were proud of her accomplishment.

The increased tendency for blacks to continue school may be due to the support of other family members. Several teenagers indicated that good jobs were scarce and the cost of child care high unless a family member or other relative was able to help.

The second pattern described by the data was teenagers' cultural response to pregnancy with respect to marriage. Among white girls there was a tendency to see marriage as the best solution to an unwanted pregnancy. Although more white girls than black girls were married at the time of an early pregnancy, all those white girls who were not married either married very soon after the discovery of the pregnancy or chose to have the baby adopted. There were no white females who were still single at the time of the interview. The above in no way suggests that the white females were in a better position to marry when they discovered they were pregnant. Rather, it suggests certain social norms regarding an unmarried woman and a child. The reactions of Patti Davis when she became pregnant at 16 give some insight to the problem-solving strategy of a white female adolescent.

Patti and her boyfriend, with whom she had been "going steady" since she was 11 years old, both had been raised in a children's home. The only difference between the two of them, as Patti described it, was that Ted was an orphan whose parents had died in an automobile accident when he was very young. Her parents were living but were unable to care for her. Ted's parents had left him a substantial amount of money that would be his at the age of 18 if he did not marry before that time.

Patti and Ted had been having unprotected intercourse since she was 13 years old. When she discovered her pregnancy, she got absolutely no support from her boyfriend. Ted's reaction was, "Have an abortion—do something to get rid of it." He obviously had no intention of jeopardizing his inheritance.

At this point Patti had nowhere to turn. She had to leave the home because she was pregnant, and she had no other family on whom she could rely. Finally a friend took her in. Jean said that Patti could stay with her as long as she needed to. In time Jean introduced

Patti to her unmarried brother, Jack. Jack, four years Patti's senior, felt sorry for her and asked her to marry him. Patti thought about his offer for several days because she was concerned that he might not know what he was doing. However, she also realized that her alternatives were limited. She told the interviewer that she had always thought love grew on you. She decided that the risk was worth it, and she married Jack. At the time of the interview Patti indicated that Jack planned to adopt her little daughter. The issue of how the child would be told her real parentage remained unsolved.

While Patti's story is admittedly unusual, it is striking testimony to the strong need of a white girl to be married when she bears a child.

On the other hand, in interview after interview black teenagers said that they hoped to be married one day, but that they were not going to rush into it before they were ready. Martha Maxwell was upset when she first discovered she was pregnant. She had thought about the risks of unprotected intercourse seriously and had been taking birth control pills regularly. (What was not clear from our interviews was whether Martha had skipped several pills and therefore exposed herself to an unexpected pregnancy, or whether she was one of those very few women who will become pregnant while taking the birth control pill regularly.) She first told her boyfriend. They talked about it for quite a while, wondering what they should do. Finally they agreed that Martha should have the baby.

Those initial discussions of what to do involved little or no mention of marriage. Martha told the interviewer a year after her baby was born that she felt she had tested her relationship with Raymond. Only then could she decide to get married. This pattern of "making sure" occurred frequently among blacks interviewed.

Francine Jones talked at length to the interviewer about her reasons for not wanting to rush into marriage. Her boyfriend, Johnny, the father of her two-year-old son, has asked her to marry him several times. So far, each time Francine had "chickened out." To her marriage was a very threatening word.

"I don't know why. I guess there's not too many that work. Sometimes they flop. I want mine to have a daddy. Some of them work. It's not all of them that flop," commented Francine thoughtfully. She continued thinking aloud, telling the interviewer that living together would be less threatening than marriage, but she did not feel she could do that because it would upset her mother too much.

"But you know marriage is hard, because it's leaving home and you're on your own. You gotta make your own decisions. When I got pregnant, my mama could help me, but if I get married, my mama will tell me, 'You go live your own life,'" continued Francine.

For Francine having a child was another step in life. But it did not carry with it a sense of total breaking with family that marriage did. As long as one only had a child, it was acceptable to remain at home and rely on one's mother for support. However, marriage, in this social structure, indicated a clear break of that family bond. You belonged with someone else. The decisions that had to be made were made by you and your spouse. In the context in which the interviewer was raised, these words to not seem at all out of place or threatening. However, within the cultural context of the black adolescent female, these words were very threatening. A black girl who decided to marry seemed put in a position of choosing between her mother and a husband. While there obviously were many things that the husband could provide that a mother could not, a mother was always there when you needed her. In this cultural context you could not always guarantee the same from a husband.

These differences in responses to an unexpected pregnancy were the main distinctions between white and black girls' handling of that situation.

APPENDIX E:
SOUTHERN CITY HEALTH DEPARTMENT
FAMILY PLANNING PAMPHLET

If you are pregnant and feel you are not ready for a baby now, there are several possibilities you can consider. We have enclosed information on maternity homes, adoption, and abortion for you to think about. It is very helpful for a woman who is considering what to do about an unwanted pregnancy to discuss her feelings with someone and to receive correct information on the kinds of help available. When you receive the results of your pregnancy test, you will be referred to a counselor who will help you with these needs. Some of the places your counselor may refer you to for help are listed on the following sheets.

If you are not pregnant and do not want a baby at this time, it is important that you obtain a good method of birth control and use it correctly. We have attached a pamphlet on family planning methods and information on where you can receive family planning aid.

FAMILY PLANNING SERVICES

1. Private physicians.

2. Southern City Health Department
   1003 Columbus Avenue
   Southern City, North Carolina

   Services include: breast and pelvic examinations; classes on methods of birth control; family planning advice; provision of birth control pills, foam, condoms; insertions of IUDs; diaphragm fitting; assistance in obtaining a tubal ligation, laparoscopy, or vasectomy. Call 000-3899 for an appointment at the family planning clinic.

3. Shadley University Infirmary. Limited to S.U. students.

4. Saint Rose College Infirmary. Limited to St. Rose students.

5. Southern City Health services. Call 000-8657 for additional information.

6. Jameson Clinic
   109 Rayburn Street
   Southern City, North Carolina

   Services include: pelvic examinations, pap smears, insertion of IUDs, prescriptions for pills, and sexual counseling. Call 000-6840 for additional information.

7. Beckett University Infirmary. Limited to Beckett students.

MATERNITY HOME INFORMATION

1. Grace Baxter Home
    Box 44
    Westbrook, North Carolina

    Charges: Based on actual cost of care and ability to pay. No woman is ever refused admission because of her inability to pay.

    Grace Baxter Home
    392 West 28th Street
    Alston, Virginia

    Grace Baxter Home
    21 East Broad Street
    Newport, Georgia

2. Baptist Children's Home
    Southern City Area Office
    12 Willow Road
    Southern City, North Carolina

    Charges: Same as above.

3. For information on North Carolina maternity home funds available to families who are unable to meet the cost of maternity home care, contact:

    Southern City Department of Social Services
    102 Pleasant Street
    Southern City, North Carolina

ORGANIZATIONS OFFERING HELP
IN PUTTING A BABY UP FOR ADOPTION

1. Southern City Department of Social Services
    102 Pleasant Street
    Southern City, North Carolina

2. Family Service—Travelers Aid Association
    139 St. James Street
    Southern City, North Carolina

3. Catholic Social Services
    777 New Hope Avenue
    Southern City, North Carolina

4. Birthchoice
    000-9346

5. Children's Home Society of North Carolina
    Box 280
    Johnson City, North Carolina

ABORTION INFORMATION

Southern City Facilities

1. Private physician, Southern City area, referred by Health Department.

   Services include: D&E, up to 12 weeks pregnant.

   Charges: $300 and up; prepayment usually required; personal check not usually accepted.

2. Southern City Memorial Hospital, outpatient clinic, appointment must be made through Health Department.

   Services include: D&E, up to 12 weeks pregnant.

   Charges: Southern City residents only, based on financial eligibility: $140 doctor fee, $200 hospital fee, $60 anesthesia, $58 RhoGram (if needed). Medicaid stickers accepted; payments arranged.

3. Jameson Center
   993 Hudson Drive
   Southern City, North Carolina

   Services include: D&E, up to 12 weeks pregnant.

   Charges: $225; prepayment required; personal checks and Medicaid stickers not accepted.

Other North Carolina Facilities

4. Dr. Hugh Smith
   Beachville, North Carolina

   Services include: Saline, up to 22 weeks pregnant.

   Charges: $340 plus $200 hospital fee; will accept Medicaid stickers.

5. Planned Parenthood of New Town
   698 Greeley Boulevard
   New Town, North Carolina

   Services include: D&E, up to 12 weeks pregnant. Must be accompanied by friend or relative.

   Charges: $150; cash; personal check not accepted; RhoGam included (cost varies).

6. Henderson Pregnancy Termination Clinic
   590 Oak Drive
   Westwood, North Carolina

   Services include: D&E, up to 12 weeks pregnant. Wednesday and Saturdays only.

   Charges: $185; cash; personal check not accepted.

7. Women's Center
   5812 Slocum Boulevard
   Lake City, North Carolina

   Services include: D&E up to 12 weeks; D&C 12 to 14 weeks (done in hospital); saline 15 to 20 weeks (done in hospital).

   Charges: $200 (depends on hospital stay); cash, money order, travelers check; no personal check.

You may obtain a pelvic examination and a physician's statement verifying uterine size by calling the family planning office at the Health Department for an appointment (000-6829). It is necessary to have a checkup two to three weeks after your abortion. You may be checked at the Health Department and enroll in the family planning clinic at the same time. Call the family planning office after your abortion for a postabortion examination.

APPENDIX F:
CHARACTERISTICS OF
WOMEN RECEIVING ABORTIONS IN
NORTH CAROLINA, 1967–76

TABLE F.1

Percentage Distribution of Abortions in North Carolina, 1967–76

	1967–1971	1972	1973	1974	1975	1976
Residence						
In state	99.2	100.0	99.3	94.0	93.2	93.5
Out of state	0.8	0.0	0.5	5.6	6.1	6.2
Age						
19 and under	30.8	36.4	34.4	37.5	37.4	36.2
20 to 29	47.2	42.9	44.8	45.6	46.6	49.7
30 and over	22.0	19.5	19.1	16.6	15.7	13.9
Mean	24.0	23.4	23.4	23.0	22.8	22.8
Race						
White	74.0	67.2	64.3	66.5	66.0	63.5
Black/other	25.6	32.6	35.5	32.6	32.8	35.3
Marital status						
Married	40.6	34.6	35.0	31.6	29.4	27.3
Unmarried	59.1	65.2	64.9	67.3	68.8	71.3
Education						
11 and under	20.0	27.0	27.5	22.6	23.2	21.1
12	23.2	31.5	32.5	27.9	29.2	28.4
13 and over	21.7	19.4	17.2	17.3	21.5	24.3
Mean	12.2	11.8	11.8	11.8	12.0	12.2
Number of living children						
None	49.6	47.2	45.0	50.6	52.4	51.7
1	13.6	15.2	17.1	17.0	18.5	20.3
2 or more	34.5	31.1	31.9	27.6	24.4	22.9
Mean	1.2	1.2	1.2	1.0	0.9	0.9
Sterilization						
Yes	15.0	12.3	12.5	7.7	7.0	7.2
No	84.9	87.4	87.0	91.8	92.4	92.7
Weeks Pregnant						
12 and under	61.6	68.6	68.9	77.7	79.0	81.8
13 to 15	15.2	12.0	10.1	7.0	7.5	6.5
16 to 20	15.9	13.2	11.6	7.1	6.4	5.9
21 and over	3.5	2.0	2.2	1.1	1.2	0.9
Mean	12.1	11.1	11.0	10.0	10.0	9.9
Operational procedure						
D&C	29.1	17.9	12.9	8.8	3.7	5.3
Suction	35.1	56.1	64.0	75.9	82.8	76.5
Saline	17.5	15.9	14.7	8.0	7.3	5.9
Hysterectomy	5.1	3.4	3.4	1.7	0.9	0.5
Hysterotomy	4.6	2.7	1.8	1.2	0.6	0.3
Prostaglandin	0.0	3.6	2.8	1.5	2.4	2.4
Other/combination	8.5	0.1	0.1	2.6	1.9	9.1

Note: Percentages may not add to 100 percent due to incomplete responses. Reporting from 1967 through May 1971 was voluntary.

Source: North Carolina Department of Human Resources, Division of Health Services, Public Health Statistics Branch, North Carolina Reported Abortions 1976.

BIBLIOGRAPHY

Abernathy, Virginia D. 1976. "Prevention of Unwanted Pregnancy among Teenagers." Primary Care 3: 399-406.

Adams, Barbara N., Carol Brownstein, Ivy M. Rennalls, and Madeline H. Schmitt. 1976. "The Pregnant Adolescent—A Group Approach." Adolescence 11: 467-85.

Alan Guttmacher Institute. 1976. 11 Million Teenagers: What Can Be Done About the Epidemic of Adolescent Pregnancies in the United States. New York: Alan Guttmacher Institute.

Badger, Earladeen, Donna Burnes, and Belinda Rhoads. 1976. "Education for Adolescent Mothers in a Hospital Setting." American Journal of Public Health 66: 469-72.

Baldwin, Wendy Harmer. 1976. "Adolescent Pregnancy and Childbearing: Growing Concerns for Americans." Population Bulletin, vol. 31 (September).

Barglow, Peter D. 1976. "Abortion in 1975: The Psychiatric Perspective, with a Discussion of Abortion and Contraception in Adolescence." Journal of Obstetric, Gynecologic and Neonatal Nursing 5: 41-48.

Braen, Bernard B., Janet Bell Forbush. 1975. "School-Age Parenthood—A National Overview." Journal of School Health 45: 256-62.

Cobliner, W. Godfrey. 1971. "Pregnancy in the Single Adolescent Girl: The Role of Cognitive Functions." Journal of Youth and Adolescence 3: 17-29.

Child Welfare League of America, Consortium on Early Childbearing and Childrearing. 1974. Adolescent Sexuality and Family Planning, an Annotated Bibliography. Washington, D.C.: National Center for Family Planning Services.

Davis, Kingsley. 1977. "The Theory of Teenage Pregnancy in the United States." Results of Current Research in Demography. International Population and Urban Research. Preliminary paper no. 10. Institute of International Studies, University of California at Berkeley.

Duenhoelter, Johann H. , Juan M. Jimines, and Gabrielle Baumann. 1975. "Pregnancy Performance of Patients under Fifteen Years of Age." Obstetrics and Gynecology 46: 49-52.

Evans, Jerome R. , Georgiana Selstad, and Wayne H. Welcher. 1976. "Teenagers: Fertility Control Behavior and Attitudes before and after Abortion, Childbearing, or Negative Pregnancy Test." Family Planning Perspectives 8: 192-200.

Foltz, Anne-Marie, Lorraine V. Klerman, and James F. Jekel. 1972. "Pregnancy and Special Education: Who Stays in School?" American Journal of Public Health 62: 1612-19.

Foster, Sallie. 1972. "Pregnancy among School-Aged Girls: A Local Evaluation of a National Problem." Public Welfare 30: 8-13.

Furstenberg, Frank F. , Jr. 1976. Unplanned Parenthood: The Social Consequences of Teenage Childbearing. New York: Free Press.

Furstenberg, Frank F. , Jr. , G. S. Masnick, and Susan A. Ricketts. 1972. "How Can Family Planning Programs Delay Repeat Teenage Pregnancies?" Family Planning Perspectives 4: 54-60.

Gabbard, Glen O. , and John R. Wolff. 1977. "The Unwed Pregnant Teenager and Her Male Relationship." Journal of Reproductive Medicine 19: 137-40.

Gedan, Sharon. 1974. "Abortion Counseling with Adolescents." American Journal of Nursing 74: 1856-58.

Gibbs, Richard F. 1973. "Therapeutic Abortion and the Minor." Journal of Legal Medicine 1: 36-42.

Gispert, Maria, and Ruth Faulk. 1976. "Sexual Experimentation and Pregnancy in Young Black Adolescents." American Journal of Obstetrics and Gynecology 126: 459-66.

Goldstein, Hyman, and Helen M. Wallace. 1978. "Services for and Needs of Pregnant Teenagers in Large Cities of the United States, 1976." Public Health Reports 93: 46-54.

Gordis, Leon, Ruth Finkelstein, and Jacqueline D. Fassett. 1970. "Evaluation of a Program for Preventing Adolescent Pregnancy." New England Journal of Medicine 282: 1078-81.

Green, Cynthia P., and Susan J. Lowe. 1975. "Teenage Pregnancy: A Major Problem for Minors." National Reporter 7: 4-5.

Gross, Ruth T., C. J. Wellington, Judith R. Williams, and E. Karayannakou. 1969. "Two Years of Experience with a Multiservice Program for Pregnant School Girls." American Public Health Association Annual Meeting . . . 1969; Collected Papers. Philadelphia: APHA.

Hartman, Evelyn. 1970. "Involvement of a Maternity and Infant Care Project in a Pregnant School Girl Program in Minneapolis, Minnesota." Journal of School Health 40: 224-27.

Haskin, Joan, Nathalie R. Hawley, and Janet B. Weinberger. 1976. "Project Teen Concern: An Educational Approach to the Prevention of Venereal Disease and Premature Parenthood." Journal of School Health 46: 231-34.

Hatcher, Sherry L. 1976. "Understanding Adolescent Pregnancy and Abortion." Primary Care 3: 407-25.

Hinman, Alan R., George Stroh, Jr., Melita C. Gesche, and Kenneth F. Whitaker. 1975. "Medical Consequences of Teenage Sexuality." New York State Journal of Medicine 75: 1439-42.

Howard, Marion. 1975. Only Human: Teenage Pregnancy and Parenthood. New York: Seabury Press.

Hunt, Williams Burr, II. 1976. Adolescent Fertility: Risks and Consequences. Population Report Series J: Family Planning Programs, no. 10. Washington, D.C.: Population Information Program, Johns Hopkins University, pp. 157-75.

Inman, Merilee. 1974. "What Teenagers Want in Sex Education." American Journal of Nursing 74: 1866-67.

International Planned Parenthood Federation. 1977. Adolescent Fertility. IPPF Bibliography Series no. 45. London: International Planned Parenthood Federation.

Jaffe, Fredericks S., and Joy G. Dryfoos. 1976. "Fertility Control Services for Adolescents: Access and Utilization." Family Planning Perspectives 8: 167-75.

Jarvis, D. L. 1972. "Preventing Illegitimate Teenage Pregnancy through Systems Interaction." Child Welfare 51: 396-401.

Jekel, James F., Jean T. Harrison, D. R. E. Bancroft, Natalie C. Tyler, and Lorraine V. Klerman. 1975. "A Comparison of the Health of Index and Subsequent Babies Born to School Age Mothers." American Journal of Public Health 65: 370-74.

Jenkins, Dorothy M. 1976. "Helping the Community Accept Human Sexuality Content in a High School Curriculum: The Case of Pomona." Journal of School Health 46: 49-50.

Johnson, Clara L. 1974. "Adolescent Pregnancy: Intervention into the Poverty Cycle." Adolescence 9: 391-406.

Jorgenson, Valerie. 1976. "Selection and Management of Contraceptives in the Adolescent Patient." Fertility and Sterility 27: 881-85.

Kinch, Robert A. H., and Elena Kruger. 1970. "Some Sociomedical Aspects of the Adolescent Pregnancy." International Journal of Gynaecology and Obstetrics 8: 480-86.

Klein, Luella. 1974. "Early Teenage Pregnancy, Contraception, and Repeat Pregnancy." American Journal of Obstetrics and Gynecology 120: 249-56.

Klerman, Lorraine V. "Adolescent Pregnancy: The Need for New Policies and New Programs." Journal of School Health 45: 263-67.

Kruger, W. Stanley. 1975. "Education for Parenthood and School-Age Parents." Journal of School Health 45: 292-95.

Lee, Luke T., and John M. Paxman. 1974/75. "Pregnancy and Abortion in Adolescence: A Comparative Legal Survey and Proposals for Reform." Columbia Human Rights Law Review 6: 307-55.

Lindemann, Constance. 1974. Birth Control and Unmarried Young Women. New York: Springer.

Lorenzi, M. Elizabeth, Lorraine V. Klerman, and James F. Jekel. 1977. "School-Age Parents: How Permanent a Relationship?" Adolescence 12: 13-22.

Menken, Jane A. 1972. "Health and Social Consequences of Teenage Childbearing." Family Planning Perspectives 4: 45-53.

Middleman, Ruth R. 1970. "A Service Pattern for Helping Unmarried Pregnant Teenagers." Children 17: 108-12.

Moore, Kristin A., and Linda J. Waite. 1977. "Early Childbearing and Educational Attainment." Family Planning Perspectives 9: 220-25.

Moore, Kristin A., and Steven B. Caldwell. 1977. "The Effect of Government Policies on Out-of-Wedlock Sex and Pregnancy." Family Planning Perspectives 9: 164-69.

Paul, Eve W., Harriet F. Pilpel, and Nancy F. Wechsler. 1976. "Pregnancy, Teenagers and the Law, 1976." Family Planning Perspectives 8: 16-21.

Perkins, Barbara Bridgman. 1974. Prevention of Adolescent Pregnancy: A Consideration of Adolescent Sexuality. Washington, D.C.: Consortium on Early Childbearing and Childrearing, Child Welfare League of America.

Redman, Linda J., and E. James Lieberman. 1973. "Abortion, Contraception and Child Mental Health." Family Planning Perspectives 5: 71-72.

Reichelt, Paul A., and Harriet H. Werley. 1975. "A Sex Information Program for Sexually Active Teenagers." Journal of School Health 45: 100-7.

Sex Information and Education Council of the United States. 1971. Teenage Pregnancy: Prevention and Treatment. Study Guide no. 14. New York: SIECUS.

Shah, Farida, Melvin Zelnik, and John F. Kantner. 1975. "Unprotected Intercourse among Unwed Teenagers." Family Planning Perspectives 7: 39-44.

Sharpe, Ruth. 1975. "Counseling Services for School-Age Pregnant Girls." Journal of School Health 45: 284-85.

Stewart, Karen Robb. 1975. Adolescent Sexuality and Teenage Pregnancy: A Selected Annotated Bibliography with Summary Forewords. Chapel Hill: State Services Office, Carolina Population Center, University of North Carolina at Chapel Hill. We found this to be an especially well done and useful bibliography.

Trussell, T. James. 1976. "Economic Consequences of Teenage Childbearing." Family Planning Perspectives 8: 184-90.

Turnbull, Craig D., and Leslie C. de Haseth. 1977. "Teenage Pregnancy in North Carolina: A 10-Year Study." North Carolina Medical Journal 38: 701-6.

University of North Carolina at Chapel Hill, Carolina Population Center Library. 1978. Consequences of Adolescent Pregnancy. PopScan Bibliography no. 311. Chapel Hill: Carolina Population Center, University of North Carolina at Chapel Hill.

Urban and Rural Systems Associates. 1976. Improving Family Planning Services for Teenagers; Final Report. Washington, D.C.: Department of Health, Education and Welfare.

Ventura, Stephanie J. 1977. "Teenage Childbearing: United States, 1966-75." Monthly Vital Statistics Report 26 (5, supp.).

Wallace, Helen M., Edwin M. Gold, Hyman Goldstein, and Allan C. Oglesby. "A Study of Services and Needs of Teenage Pregnant Girls in the Large Cities of the United States." American Journal of Public Health 63: 5-16.

Whelan, Elizabeth Murphy, and George K. Higgins. 1973. Teenage Childbearing: Extent and Consequences. Washington, D.C.: Consortium on Early Childbearing and Childrearing, Child Welfare League of America.

Zelnik, Melvin, and John F. Kantner. 1978. "First Pregnancies to Women Aged 15 to 19: 1976 and 1971." Family Planning Perspectives 10: 11-20.

_____. 1975. "Attitudes of American Teenagers toward Abortion." Family Planning Perspectives 7: 89-91.

Zongker, Calvin E. 1977. "The Self Concept of Pregnant Adolescent Girls." Adolescence 12: 477-88.

abortion, 85, 127; access to, 85;
attitudes toward, 25, 107-26;
characteristics of opposers, 113-
17, 121-26; clinics, 85-88, 90,
91-92; composite abortion attitude
scale, 111-13; cost of, 87, 88,
90, 105-7; decision frame, 24,
47-48; demographic influence of,
113-17, 121; in Farmville, 88,
89-90; funding for, 15-16; geographical spread of, 85-88; hospital role in, 31, 85-89; illegal,
48, 88; parental consent requirement for, 119-26; policies, 16,
89-90; proportion to teenagers,
97-101; rates [Farmville, 88;
health systems area, 101; North
Carolina, 12-15, 101; Southern
City, 88; United States, 15, 102-
5]; ratios, 102-5; respondents'
views on [acceptability of, 111-13,
117-19, 126, 163-68; availability,
85, 85-93, 130, 132-33, 135; program funding for, 163-68; without
parental consent, 119-26]; as sex
education topic, 191-93; in Southern City, 88, 91-105; unmet need
for, 102-7
adolescent development as sex education topic, 187-88, 189, 190-93
adoption: agency roles in counseling pregnant teens about, 67, 71,
84; as option chosen by teenagers,
68, 75
adults as counselors, 31
Aid to Families with Dependent
Children (AFDC), 195, 222
American Public Health Association (APHA), 2-3, 5; policies,
22, 239-41

birth control (see contraceptive
programs; contraceptives)
birthrates (see fertility)
birth statistics, U.S., 10-12;
(see also North Carolina)
blacks, 8 (see also racial differences)
boyfriend (see father, biological)

churches (see ministers; religion)
city councilmen: recommendations of, 217-19; views on [abor-
tion, 88; pregnancy counseling,
84; pregnancy testing, 84]
community leaders (see influentials)
community services (see abortion;
contraceptive programs; counseling; family planning programs;
Health Department; hotline; pregnancy testing; and sex education)
condoms, 151-52
confidants, 25-26, 31-51; respondents' views on, 27-31, 50-51
confidentiality, 220
Congress, U.S.: sample characteristics, 18; views on [abor-
tion 117-19, 126-27, 168; contraceptive services, 159-68;
counseling pregnant teens, 84;
pregnancy testing, 77, 84; sex
education, 200]
contraceptive methods, sources
of, 149-53; pharmacists, 133-
34; physicians, 130, 133; Public
Health Department, 130
contraceptive programs, 128-73;
availability to teens, 129-30,
135-36, 232; barriers to use, 137-
38; clinic procedures in, 141-42;

ABOUT THE AUTHORS

JAMES E. ALLEN is an Associate Professor in the Department of Health Administration in the School of Public Health and Senior Research Associate at the Carolina Population Center, University of North Carolina at Chapel Hill. He holds a B.A. from the University of Arizona (1957) and the S.T.M. degree (1960) and Ph.D. degree (1964) in sociology and ethics from Boston University. In addition he holds the M.S.P.H. degree (1968) from the University of North Carolina at Chapel Hill. Publications include over 20 articles, an earlier book, and a monograph in the field of population program management.

Since 1968 he has conducted research projects under grants from the Ford Foundation, the Agency for International Development, and the National Institute for Child and Human Development. Dr. Allen also has served as a population consultant to the Ford Foundation, Department of Health, Education and Welfare, and the Center for Family Planning Program Development (now the Alan Guttmacher Institute). He served for four years on the board of directors of Planned Parenthood of Massachusetts and for three years on the board of directors of Planned Parenthood of Iowa. Currently he is an active member of a North Carolina state government task force studying adolescent fertility problems in that state.

DEBORAH BENDER is a clinical instructor and Associate Director of the Off-Campus Master's Degree Program in the Department of Health Administration at Chapel Hill.

She holds a B.A. from Boston College (Newton Campus, 1969) and is completing her doctoral dissertation in medical anthropology at the American University in Washington, D.C.

Her past experience includes educational program development for children and research in Himba (Angola), population migration patterns at the Smithsonian Institution, and teaching at Washington International College—a community institution for experience-based education.

She has conducted field research on patient satisfaction with health care in urban health clinics, in cooperation with the District of Columbia Public Interest Research Group (PIRG). She is presently a member of the Orange County Task Force on Adolescent Health, which is working to develop and coordinate community services for teenagers.